Martin E. Goldman, M.D., F.A.A.C.

The Handbook of

....

Heart
Drugs

A Consumer's Guide to Safe
and Effective Use

Henry Holt and Company
New York

Published by Henry Holt and Company, Inc.,
115 West 18th Street, New York, New York 10011.
Published in Canada by Fitzhenry & Whiteside Limited,
91 Granton Drive, Richmond Hill, Ontario, L4B 2N5.

Library of Congress Cataloging-in-Publication Data
Goldman, Martin E.
The handbook of heart drugs : a consumer's guide to safe and
effective use / Martin E. Goldman.—1st ed.
p.   cm.
"An Owl book."
1. Cardiovascular agents—Handbooks, manuals, etc.
2. Cardiovascular agents—Popular works.   I. Title.
RM345.G635   1992   91-39966
615'71—dc20   CIP
ISBN 0-8050-1720-8
ISBN 0-8050-1721-6 (An Owl book: pbk.)

Henry Holt books are available at special discounts
for bulk purchases for sales promotions, premiums,
fund-raising, or educational use. Special editions
or book excerpts can also be created to specification.
For details contact: Director, Special Markets.

First Edition—1992

Illustrations by Nancy Kriebel
Printed in the United States of America
Recognizing the importance of preserving the written word,
Henry Holt and Company, Inc., by policy, prints all of its
first editions on acid-free paper. ∞

3   5   7   9   10   8   6   4   2

3   5   7   9   10   8   6   4   2
pbk.

*The information in this book was designed to educate individuals on some of the effects
and uses of heart medication. It is in no way meant as a substitute for regular medical
care. The author strongly recommends that the drugs profiled herein be used only under
the supervision of a cardiologist or other medical doctor.*

To the memory of my beloved mother,
Shirley Shifra Goldman,
and in honor of her granddaughter,
Sarah Shifra,
who bears her name.

Acknowledgments

This book represents a culmination of a personal education that began as a child: by my mother, Shirley, a woman of valor and an educator of emotionally disturbed children who instilled in me a passion for life and an empathy for all people; by my father, Hirsh, who exemplified dedication, responsibility, and personal interactive skills as a pharmacist for over sixty years; by my uncle Solomon Goldman, M.D., a dermatologist for over fifty years, who loved the practice of medicine.

My education at Yeshiva University inculcated me with the importance of a moral and holistic approach to people and their sufferings. An internship and residency at Peter Bent Brigham of Harvard University in Boston and a cardiology fellowship at Mount Sinai in New York provided me with a solid foundation in medicine and important role models, including Eugene Braunwald, M.D., Simon Dack, M.D., Valentin Fuster, M.D., Richard Gorlin, M.D., Jose Meller, M.D., Bruce Mindich, M.D., and Marshal Wolf, M.D.

I would like to express my heartfelt appreciation to John Gallagher, without whom this book would not have been possible. I would also like to thank my editor at Henry Holt, Theresa Burns, whose editorial patience and skills were greatly appreciated, especially at those moments when we faced knotty problems of organization and approach. I'd also like to thank Nancy Kriebel for providing illustrations to the book.

Finally, I express my deepest gratitude to my co-workers and patients who continue to teach me about medicine and life every day.

Contents

Contents

PART TWO
Cardiovascular Drug Profiles

List of Heart Drugs

DIURETICS

THIAZIDE-TYPE DIURETICS

Brand Name	Generic Name
HYDRODIURIL, ESIDRIX, ORETIC, THIURETIC, MICTRIN	hydrochlorothiazide
ZAROXOLYN, DIULO, MYKROX	metolazone
LOZOL	indapamide

LOOP DIURETICS

Brand Name	Generic Name
LASIX, AGRO-FUROSEMIDE, MYROSEMIDE	furosemide
BUMEX	bumetanide

POTASSIUM-SPARING DIURETICS

Brand Name	Generic Name
ALDACTONE	spironolactone
MIDAMOR	amiloride hydrochloride
DYRENIUM	triamterene

DIURETIC COMBINATIONS

Brand Name	*Generic Name*
DYAZIDE	triamterene and hydro-chlorothiazide
MAXZIDE	triamterene and hydro-chlorothiazide
MODURETIC	amiloride hydrochloride and hydrochlorothiazide

BETA BLOCKERS

B1-SELECTIVE BETA-ADRENERGIC BLOCKERS

Brand Name	*Generic Name*
LOPRESSOR	metoprolol
TENORMIN	atenolol

NONSELECTIVE BETA-ADRENERGIC BLOCKERS

Brand Name	*Generic Name*
BLOCADREN	timolol maleate
INDERAL, INDERAL LA	propranolol hydro-chloride
SECTRAL	acebutolol hydrochloride
CORGARD	nadolol
VISKEN	pindolol
LEVATOL	penbatolol sulfate
CARTROL	carteolol hydrochloride
KERLONE	betaxolol

ALPHA- AND BETA-ADRENERGIC BLOCKERS

Brand Name	*Generic Name*
NORMODYNE, TRANDATE	labetalol hydrochloride

CALCIUM ANTAGONISTS (CALCIUM CHANNEL BLOCKERS)

Brand Name	*Generic Name*
CALAN, CALAN SR, ISOPTIN, ISOPTIN SR	verapamil hydrochloride
PROCARDIA	nifedipine
CARDIZEM, CARDIZEM SR	diltiazem hydrochloride

VASODILATORS

PERIPHERAL VASODILATORS

Brand Name	*Generic Name*
APRESOLINE, HYDRALAZINE HCI	hydralazine hydrochloride

ALPHA-1-ADRENERGIC BLOCKERS

Brand Name	*Generic Name*
MINIPRESS	prazosin hydrochloride
HYTRIN	terazosin hydrochloride

ANGIOTENSIN-CONVERTING ENZYME (ACE) INHIBITORS

Brand Name	*Generic Name*
CAPOTEN	captopril
VASOTEC	enalapril maleate

NITRATES

Brand Name	Generic Name
NIPRIDE, NITROPRESS	sodium nitroprusside
LONITEN	minoxidil

CENTRAL ALPHA-ADRENERGIC AGONISTS

Brand Name	Generic Name
ALDOMET	methyldopa
CATAPRES	clonidine
WYTENSIN	guanabenz acetate
TENEX	guanfacine hydrochloride

PERIPHERAL ADRENERGIC BLOCKERS

Brand Name	Generic Name
SERPASIL, SERPALAN	reserpine
HYLOREL	guanadrel sulfate
ISMELIN	guanethidine monosulfate

POTASSIUM SUPPLEMENTS

Brand Name	Generic Name
K-DUR	potassium chloride
K-LOR, K-LYTE/CL, KAOCHLOR, KAON-CL, KATO, KLORVESS, KLOTRIX, K-TAB, MICRO-K LS, EXTENCAPS, SK-POTASSIUM CHLORIDE, SLOW-K, TEN-K	potassium bicarbonate
K-LYTE, K-LYTE DS	potassium bicarbonate

ANTIARRHYTHMICS

Brand Name	Generic Name
LANOXIN, LANOXICAPS	digoxin
NORPACE	disopyramide phosphate
PROCAN SR, PROMINE, PRONESTYL, PRONESTYL-SR	procainamide hydrochloride
QUINAGLUTE DURA-TABS, DURAQUIN, QUINALAN	quinidine gluconate
CINQUIN, QUINIDEX EXTENTABS, QUINORA	quinidine sulfate
CARDIOQUIN	quinidine polygalacturonate
TAMBOCOR	flecainide acetate
MEXITIL	mexiletine hydrochloride
CORDARONE	amiodarone

BLOOD-RELATED DRUGS

ANTICOAGULANT AGENTS

Brand Name	Generic Name
COUMADIN	warfarin sodium
HEPARIN, LIQUAEMIN	heparin sodium

THROMBOLYTIC AGENTS

Brand Name	Generic Name
KABIKINASE, STREPTASE	streptokinase
ACTIVASE	alteplase, recombinant

HEMORHEOLOGIC AGENTS

Brand Name	*Generic Name*
TRENTAL	pentoxifylline

ANTIPLATELET AGENTS

Brand Name	*Generic Name*
PERSANTINE, PYRIDAMOLE	dipyridamole
BUFFERIN and many other aspirin-containing medications	acetylsalicylic acid

ANTIHYPERLIPIDEMICS

Brand Name	*Generic Name*
QUESTRAN	cholestyramine
COLESTID	colestipol
ATROMID-S	clofibrate
LOPID	gemfibrozil
MEVACOR	lovastatin
NICOLAR	niacin or nicotinic acid
LORELCO	probucol
CHOLOXIN	dextrothyroxine

Introduction

Each year approximately 400,000 people die suddenly of cardiac abnormalities—primarily coronary artery disease—some congenital, others acquired valvular disease. These deaths occur not only among people who have been treated for heart disease but also among seemingly healthy people, even superb athletes such as college basketball players or Olympic volleyball players.

Yet, as disturbing as these figures are, the number of deaths related to coronary disease has actually *declined* about 25 percent in the last decade. Superior medical care of heart attack victims—by both emergency medical services and intensive-care units—has allowed many more people to survive heart attacks. New procedures for acute heart attack victims, such as angioplasty—which opens up blocked blood vessels and immediately improves blood flow—have saved many lives. We have also reduced the severity and number of heart attacks in this country by more effectively treating hypertension and diabetes, by recognizing the risk posed by a family history of heart disease, and by reducing or modifying specific risk factors, such as cigarette smoking and high-fat diets.

But what may be the most decisive factor in our growing success in the treatment of heart disease has been the introduction of new drugs. The approach to cardiac disease from a pharmacological point of view has dramatically changed in the last ten years and certainly is drastically different from the approach of the early 1970s. A large number of heart drugs profiled in this book were not available as recently as twenty years ago, and some as recently as ten and five years ago. Prior to that time we had fewer diuretics, only a limited number of arrhythmics, and no selective beta blockers or calcium channel blockers. With the arrival of these newer drugs, we have been able not only to save many lives but also to prevent a recurrence of the heart disease, and at the same time to reduce the side effects and general inconveniences associated with drug therapy.

Although we would like heart drugs to affect only the cardiovascular system, specifically the heart or blood vessels, they inevitably affect other systems in the body, such as the liver, the lungs, and the brain. In the past, for instance, some patients who took beta blockers to treat their angina at times found it difficult to breathe, especially if they had a history of asthma. In the past few years, however, new *selective* beta blockers have been introduced that are capable of eliminating those side effects by restricting their effects to just the heart and coronary arteries.

New drugs have also brought about radical changes in the emergency-room treatment of people who have had heart attacks. Patients today have a far greater chance to survive a heart attack because immediate treatment with medications can dissolve the blood clots that caused the heart attack in the first place. Also, the recent development of a whole array of antiarrhythmic medications has proved effective in preventing sudden unexpected collapse and death from heart rhythm disturbances following a heart attack.

Another development is our improved understanding of various drug reactions. As a result, heart medications can be used more effectively. One example of this involves a blood thinner, Coumadin. Because at one time Coumadin was thought to cause excessive bleeding, the drug was seldom prescribed. But recently we have learned that at lower doses the drug can remain effective while producing relatively few side effects.

So in many ways new drugs have changed our approach to the treatment and management of cardiovascular disease—and the future may hold even more dramatic changes. It's expected that new delivery systems for medications, such as more effective external "patches," or long-acting injections under the skin, will lead to a more natural control of diseases than is possible with drugs taken intermittently. Even more important, drugs may soon be able to *reverse* much of the damage caused by heart disease, something that is beyond the capability of most current heart drugs. Dramatic changes may also occur as a result of laser technology, which allows the removal of cholesterol plaques in blood vessels before they can create problems.

I have a 2-year-old daughter, Sarah Shifra Abigail. As I watch her early development, I'm amazed at the complexity of the human body—its smooth functioning as well as its beauty and fragility. As a father and as a doctor I know how important it is that we take great pains to protect and cherish this delicate mechanism. Many people, unfortunately, fail to realize this until it is too late.

And so I find it encouraging that yet another growing trend in medicine has been the increasing number of people who each year seek the help of trained cardiologists to evaluate their potential risk for heart disease and learn about its prevention. More and more people seem to understand that the deleterious consequences of heart disease are avoidable. While this book describes in detail many of the important facts concerning the drugs that may be prescribed for you, it also places a special emphasis on how improved cardiac health can be significantly affected by a working partnership with your cardiologist.

Part 1 of this book describes all of the important issues you should be aware of *before* taking any cardiovascular medication. These chapters discuss what to look for in a cardiologist, how to enhance the value of your visits to the doctor, and how to monitor your own progress under his or her care. We will examine here the various tests and procedures used in the diagnosis and treatment of heart disease (including heart valve and bypass surgery, coronary angioplasty, and artificial pacemakers), the general nature of a number of common coronary illnesses, some considerations before making a decision to undergo surgery, and, finally, some important information about risk factors—ones we control and ones we do not—that affect heart disease.

In Part 2 of this book I profile more than ninety individual heart drugs, giving you an understanding of how each drug works, its side effects, and any potential adverse reactions. Each listing provides a brief discussion of how the drug should be taken, what foods or other drugs should be avoided while taking the drug, and what specific symptoms require your doctor's attention.

In summary, this book is addressed to you, the patient, and your family in the hope that you will be able to approach the complexities of heart disease and its treatment with greater skill and confidence. But even more important, I hope that it will help you communicate better with your physician, appreciate the rationale and therapeutic experience of your prescribed treatment, and, most of all, convince you that good medicine is the primary goal of two people—you and your doctor.

Martin E. Goldman, M.D.
March 1992

PART ONE
············

What You Should
Know Before Taking
Heart Drugs

ONE

·········

Doctor-Patient Issues

Heart disease is a very personal illness because no effective understanding of it can be expected without a detailed knowledge of the patient. The way we live our lives has a great deal to do with this illness: how it occurs and how it should be treated.

As you will see later, many heart patients share intimate and confidential information about themselves, their families, and their disease with their cardiologists. In turn, the effective physician respectfully probes into personal and professional lives, all in an effort to examine the integral bond between the stress and strains of patients' lives and the characteristics of their illnesses.

As a result, a relationship between you and your cardiologist that is trusting and personally disclosing will serve both your and your doctor's needs. You benefit because you will more likely understand and believe in the commitment demanded by treatment and recovery; your cardiologist benefits because openness usually provides the kinds of information the treatment requires.

How personal that relationship becomes depends upon your doctor's willingness to ask and your willingness to disclose. It also depends upon the nature and severity of the illness and how your own life-style affects it. But I believe that better treatment results when patients, especially those who may have cause to be fretful and worried, find that they can be safely revealing to their doctor.

Need to Disclose

Probably your relationship with your cardiologist will differ from past relationships with doctors, because this relationship involves life-and-death issues. In the case of heart disease and its potential for a sudden catastrophic event, your health care takes on a heightened sense of urgency—or at least it should.

Most people with heart disease understand, at least in theory, that they could die without prior warning, which usually makes them not only more anxious but also more vigilant. By comparison, it is unlikely that you would die suddenly as a result of an ulcer. Worse, if you had Crohn's disease, which produces abdominal cramps and bloody diarrhea, you would suffer days of genuine sickness, and your general health would be seriously affected, but you wouldn't have to worry about dying the next day. Cancer may be the most depressing disease to experience, but even cancer patients can be told of therapeutic options, though their prognosis may be poor.

With heart disease, however, many patients hear a different story. More than once I have had the unpleasant task of telling people after they had an angiogram that unless they had coronary bypass surgery, they were at significant risk of having a major heart attack or possibly dying suddenly. I did not say this to frighten them, but to alert them to the gravity of their illness. Striking this note of urgency has often set the tone for a very effective and intimate medical treatment program.

For some patients the need to be direct and candid about their private lives with a medical doctor is unfamiliar and stressful. But most people do realize it's in their best interest to trust and cooperate with their cardiologist. Unfortunately, however, I still find some patients who either do not appreciate the seriousness of their illness or outright deny that they are sick. Admittedly, disclosing certain feelings, behaviors, or circumstances of your home or business life can be difficult. It is reasonable to protect our privacy and reveal personal information only when we believe it is appropriate or necessary. It's important to recognize how heart disease can be adversely affected by our private lives. Omitting to tell your physician significant details of your disease experience can undermine your care. For example, it may be embarrassing to talk about chest pain during intercourse or an argument with your spouse or another family member. I would be embarrassed, too. But not sharing these important signs of heart disease may place you at grave risk.

Many doctors find the experience of having a noncompliant, uncooperative patient who continues to complain of symptoms frustrating and dissatisfying. If a doctor comes to believe that a patient is undermining the therapeutic regimen prescribed, the doctor, I believe, could actually become less interested in that patient's care.

All heart patients need to take an active role in the treatment of their disease: understand it and what arouses or triggers any of its symptoms; accurately report all your symptoms to your doctor; follow any instructions about diet, exercise, and medications; and especially report any unusual reactions to your drugs. To do all this, you must feel comfortable with your doctor. Think of your relationship with your cardiologist as a partnership. If one member of a partnership doesn't provide all the information needed to conduct its business, or the other is not sufficiently skilled to deal with that information, the aim of that partnership—in this case, your health care—may very well fail.

You are unique, and this fact governs how your doctor creates your treatment program. Your cardiologist will start with some initial guidelines based on knowledge of how other people in similar circumstances have responded to your disease. But this general information is inadequate to predict the course of your treatment with absolute confidence. Increasing reliability of any treatment for heart disease is dependent on the unique and characteristic data you provide the doctor. It begins with being absolutely candid about your disease during your first visit and then letting your doctor know precisely how you are responding to the treatment and medications during subsequent visits. We'll discuss the first visit in more detail later in this chapter.

The guiding principle in clinical medicine is to treat the person, not the disease, and this is especially true in cardiology. If your feedback to your doctor about yourself and your response to therapy is vague or inaccurate, it could be said that your doctor is not treating *you*, but *your disease.*

Your Attitude Toward Your Disease

It can be very important to your care for you to know what your attitude is toward your illness. Many heart patients begin therapy fearful that they may not recover. Health-care professionals believe that such attitudes strongly influence how and when the patient recovers.

After you've had your illness professionally diagnosed, there are two important areas to think about: First, how will you accept professional treatment and your patient role? Second, how will you accept your recovery and rehabilitation?

In some respects, doctor and patient are dependent on each other: You rely on the doctor for care and supervision, and the doctor depends on your input and cooperation for successful treatment. Matching yourself with the right doctor for your personality is just as important as seeking a doctor well qualified in cardiology. Some doctors demand that their patients be absolutely obedient and never deviate from their directives. Some patients find this attitude acceptable, or even preferable. Increasingly, however, patients find that an autocratic tone makes them uncomfortable. Hence, you need to know yourself well enough to realize whether working under this discipline will lead to subtle resistance on your part. If you feel that a policing attitude might cause you to rebel and not comply or to fear the doctor's disapproval were you to disobey some instructions, you should discuss this feeling openly on your first visit. You would not want to feel you had to hide from your doctor instances when you were unable to follow the regimen. You may also realize that you need a physician who spends more time discussing options and planning care rather than being dictatorial.

The second attitude concerns recovery. It's reasonable to assume that all patients want to recover, but some people struggle with the fear that they will never actually be "normal" again. It's important for patients to know in advance that they will be experiencing unfamiliar emotions and reactions. I tell my patients that following surgery they might become emotional and suddenly start to cry. Such moments can be startling, especially for someone who has seldom expressed his or her feelings. The trauma of surgery, the anxiety and sleeplessness, the effect of medications, and the general weariness all contribute to a feeling of vulnerability. Understandably, some patients come to feel they are falling apart and, worse, that they are going to die or be permanently incapacitated.

In truth, there is no way to have a heart attack and not be upset by it. But I find that many patients initially hear only the "worst-case scenario," which can cause significant anxiety and disrupt their normal life pattern. There are steps to take to minimize anxiety, anger, or depression. First, realize that they may occur. Also, understand that your recovery will take time; it will occur day by day, often more slowly than you want. You must have patience.

Everyone's recovery is different. Just because a friend or relative has had the same heart disease or surgery, it does not necessarily mean that your recovery will be similar. Your recovery depends on several factors: the extent and complications of your heart attack, the level of your activity before the heart attack, and your heart's response to increases in activity. Recovery from surgery is discussed in more detail in Chapter 5.

It's important to address fears and anxieties, because people who are constantly fearful or depressed often recover more slowly and less thoroughly. Discuss your apprehensions with your doctor, even if you think they are crazy. Some of these "crazy" thoughts may, in fact, lead your doctor to a helpful diagnosis. If your depression or anxiety continues for four weeks or more, your doctor may give you some medication or, if necessary, suggest counseling.

Your Attitude Toward Your Doctor

As discussed before, your relationship with your doctor can affect your treatment. A few years ago a colleague of mine was treating a fifty-year-old man for hypertension. Instead of taking his medications as he was instructed, the man said he took them only intermittently because they affected his libido.

Because the patient reduced the dosage of his medication, his blood pressure remained dangerously high. Believing the original dose was ineffective, his doctor increased the dosage in an effort to improve the patient's performance. This time the patient was significantly alarmed over the dangers of his hypertension and, instead of arbitrarily reducing his dosage, he faithfully and correctly took his new medications, as instructed. Within two weeks, he became gravely weak, a serious sign of a medication overdose. Once the doctor learned that the man had not been taking the earlier dosage as scheduled and that his patient was, in effect, now being overmedicated, he immediately lowered the dosage to the original dose. The patient's symptoms disappeared and his blood pressure was controlled.

Sexual issues are always difficult to talk about, especially a diminished sexual drive. But as delicate an issue as it may be to discuss, the patient should not take it upon himself to treat the problem by adjusting his own medication. Perhaps the doctor did not adequately explain the potential for this side effect, or failed to explain the seriousness of reducing the dosage. In any event, the patient so disliked his physician that he decided to take matters in his own hands rather than reveal that he had not taken the medication as directed and the reason.

8

Another issue to consider is the self-esteem of a doctor. As strange as it may seem to some patients, doctors are human and fear rejection like everyone else. If they feel rejected by uncooperative patients, or their professional integrity is challenged, it can affect the quality of care they provide. A study by a group of medical experts about doctors who had disrespectful patients revealed troubling findings: Doctors who felt resentment toward a patient could be less attentive or meticulous in their treatment.

A different study suggested that people accustomed to intimidating others by exercising their authority over them often treat their doctors in a similar manner. Out of a misguided belief that this is the way to get the best care, they actually harass and bully their doctors if dissatisfied with the care. If someone thinks he may die, this may be understandable behavior. But if someone uses such behavior merely to establish authority during routine care, it can be counterproductive.

Senior corporate executives who are always struggling for control of their business fate may have difficulty relinquishing control of their medical fate to their doctors. Regrettably, the study showed that instead of getting the best care, their bluster could be endangering their health. Experts believe that a doctor who feels intimidated may be reluctant to make health-care demands on the patient that might anger or alienate him and may actually defer tests or needed procedures.

A case in point: I have a patient who is an extremely wealthy and powerful businessman and a board member of several prominent medical schools and universities. Because he's always in a rush, people in his path suffer from his haste and sharp tongue. But he and I share a different kind of relationship. As dominating as he is in his world, he has come to understand that his health depends on my being dominant in mine. Early on, I said that if he had to hurry during our visit, he was free to leave. But I added that it would be in his best interest to sit and discuss his medical problem until he and I were both satisfied. I likened it to a business deal: I wanted to serve him as best I could so he could leave with the assurance that he would be healthy enough to keep making money. That approach appealed to him immediately. The man still storms, blusters, and boasts in his own world, but when we interact in my office at the hospital, he's utterly cooperative—almost congenially so. He uses his experience and intelligence to ask prudent questions regarding his illness or therapeutic plan rather than to exert his authority.

Private Lives

Sometimes it is difficult to be candid with your doctor; but remember, your health is far more important than any momentary embarrassment. A few years ago I had a patient with angina and a complicated story that threatened to compromise my ability to treat his heart disease. He was forty-one years old and twenty pounds overweight. He came to the emergency room because of an anginal episode. When he came back the next day for our first visit, I learned that he had been having chest pains two and three times a week for almost a month. I also learned that he had been under the care of another cardiologist for the past six months and was receiving medication from him, but was not happy with his care because he felt the doctor disliked him.

He said he had been under a lot of financial stress since he was a struggling architect in a weak economy. As we talked further, he admitted he was divorced with a fifteen-year-old daughter, whom he missed very much. He was in relatively good health and in no immediate danger of having a heart attack. However, I told him he had to reduce the stress level in his life. I also suggested some regular exercise.

It took him three visits and a catheterization (a procedure that involves passing a tube through an artery) before he told me what he believed was the principal problem related to the anginal episodes: two years earlier he had declared to his wife that he was gay, which led to the divorce. Since then he had often been lonely. But when he went to gay bars he felt more anxious and troubled because of his physical appearance. His hair was thinning and he was overweight.

His deep-seated anxiety came from his fear that he would be rejected if he told anyone he had a heart condition. "Other gay men want younger companions," he said, "not a fat old man with heart disease." His heart condition was his secret.

I subsequently learned that he had not told his other cardiologist about his personal life for fear that he would be rejected by his doctor as he had been by his mother, father, and brother. No one outside the family knew the details of his gay life-style or his heart condition. He said it was a relief to open up and tell me what was troubling him. I was sure that his disclosure was the beginning of his accepting responsibility for his health and, thus, improving the possibility of a successful outcome.

There was more to come. On his next visit he told me that he had been seeing a psychiatrist for almost two years. He felt such shame about his secret life, however, that he forbade his psychiatrist for almost a year from calling the other cardiologist and then me about the fact that she had prescribed a psychiatric drug, amitriptyline, for his depression. Since one of the potential adverse reactions of amitriptyline is a heart rhythm disturbance, the therapist was afraid that his cardiologist might treat him for these symptoms not knowing they were the side effects of the amitriptyline. But she could not compel him to tell his other cardiologist, nor could she telephone herself, as the details of his treatment with her were held in absolute confidence.

Finally he relented. The psychiatrist called me and we were able to share the information of our respective drug therapies. If she had not called and I had seen irregular heartbeats (caused by the amitriptyline), I would have stopped the drug I was giving him thinking the cardiac drug was the sole cause. This patient overcame a tremendous obstacle to divulge a very private aspect of his life. In his own words, his health improved as soon as he began "to live honestly."

11

More Than One Doctor

Many of my patients have been referred to me by another doctor, and more than a few have several doctors treating them for several different disorders. In these cases, I find it very important that my patients have one doctor who will centralize their health care and, especially, coordinate their medicines.

Frequently, patients have had extensive tests—or at least X-rays or electrocardiograms—before they see a consultant. If you can bring any prior examination results to the consulting physician, as well as a brief summary of your past treatment or a summary of your case history from your other doctor, there is a substantial savings of both time and money. The consulting physician does not have to repeat studies and previously tried unsuccessful therapies.

Sometimes having more than one doctor is helpful. One afternoon a man was admitted to the hospital with an undiagnosed heart problem. He was a minister. That morning while speaking to his congregation he had become sweaty and then very cold. It was not clear whether he had sustained a heart rhythm disturbance or a small stroke. I saw him that night and felt that the event was not cardiac in origin. The next day I sent him to a neurologist in the hospital. The minister asked me not to notify his regular internist (who was his close friend and member of his congregation) that he was consulting other doctors because, he believed, the internist would feel insulted. The next day the patient called to say that he had seen the neurologist, who told him he'd had a "ministroke" and gave him a course of management. But he still did not want to tell his internist.

I told him that seeing another doctor was not a matter of infidelity, as if he were seeing another woman. His internist and friend would probably understand and welcome the fact that he was receiving expert medical care. Moreover, his regular doctor might be eager to consult and share with me any relevant medical data. He might well benefit by having his two doctors talk to each other and pool their thoughts about his condition. Eventually he relented and I called his doctor. As I anticipated, the doctor was glad to hear that his friend was receiving expert care, and together we outlined an appropriate diagnostic and therapeutic plan based in part on his knowledge of the patient.

Selecting a Cardiologist

Most people, if asked, would say that they do not feel comfortable judging the competency of a doctor, in particular a specialist, such as a cardiologist. At the same time most people hold a relatively firm opinion on the quality of care they are receiving from their own doctor. Those two opinions are not unrelated: Care is one of the essential issues of competency.

Still, it is very difficult for a patient to know who is considered a good physician. Unfortunately, many people remain impressed with unrelated evidence, such as an expensively furnished office in a high-rent district. Even gray hair appears important to some people, as if age automatically imparts needed medical expertise.

The importance of a wise choice when selecting a personal doctor is unquestionably greater than when making a financial investment. Yet most people give more care and attention to the business of their money than the business of their medical care. We are extremely thorough before purchasing a home. We do not make this decision frivolously or impulsively, since it is a major investment that usually affects us for years to come. We also consult the opinions of others in buying a home: we are willing to take time to find the right realtor, consult with other homeowners in the neighborhood, and hire a professional appraiser, engineer, or architect to assess the value of the property.

It's my experience, however, that people do not exercise anywhere near the same care and patience in selecting a cardiologist, whose recommendations and judgments can obviously have lifelong consequences. In this age of specialized medicine, it's only

13

prudent to see a doctor who is trained to handle your specific health problem. If you have cancer, you consult a board-certified oncologist; if you have a heart condition, see a cardiologist.

A lawyer who had become very wealthy through mergers and acquisitions came to me complaining of chest pains. I learned that he had been treated by a local doctor, an internist who accepted and treated patients with heart disease but was not trained as a cardiologist. The doctor diagnosed a dangerous heart condition and insisted that the lawyer strictly refrain from any strenuous activity.

This astute businessman blindly accepted the diagnosis and treatment recommendations of a local doctor, unaware of the status of the doctor's credentials to treat a highly specialized problem. Had this lawyer been asked to purchase the office building owned by the doctor, he would have thoroughly examined the doctor's background long before he even sat down to talk to him.

The patient was devastated when the internist told him to undertake a complete change of life-style. A man who normally played two sets of tennis each week (and usually won), attended health spas periodically, and went skiing with his family every winter was told to become an invalid at the age of 52.

For four months he struggled with his new life, believing he was a very sick man. His wife, who was a patient of mine then, convinced him that it was foolish not to seek a second opinion. She called and asked me to see her husband. What I discovered was that he had a mild form of heart muscle thickness (hypertrophic cardiomyopathy) that did not call for a major life change, but did require totally different medications than he had been given. The false diagnosis probably resulted because the local doctor had seen this type of condition at most once or twice, whereas cardiologists at a major medical center have opportunities to see similar conditions more frequently. Five years later the man is in excellent health, thanks in no small part to the steady regimen of exercise he once was about to abandon.

Most patients know that selecting a cardiologist requires more than consulting the Yellow Pages. At a minimum they will ask a friend or relative for a recommendation. Unfortunately, too many people are willing to accept the very first cardiologist recommended to them, whether the suggestion came from a fellow patient or another doctor. And when they engage the services of the cardiologist, they are reluctant to express what they want in terms of their care, as if it's impertinent to discuss their reservations with a doctor.

Hiring a doctor should not be unlike doing business with other professionals: before entrusting them with your greatest asset, you need to make inquiries about their qualifications.

Before Selecting a Cardiologist

Before selecting a cardiologist, learn whether the doctor is affiliated with a major medical center. Every major city has at least one hospital that by reputation is considered "the medical center," that is, a good-sized hospital affiliated with a medical school. Doctors on staff in these hospitals usually are familiar with the latest medications, related technologies, and the professional literature of their specialties.

One question to consider is whether the doctor is a full-time employee of the university or hospital or is only part time (sometimes referred to as "voluntary"). A doctor with a full-time teaching position at the hospital is held to the highest standards of the medical center, and may be teaching or doing research as well as seeing patients. On the other hand, cardiologists who are part-time staff, or only have admitting privileges, are able to treat their own patients in the hospital, i.e., these doctors have met the *general* standards demanded by that institution. Thus, some "private" physicians may be superb clinicians while others may not be.

Physicians who are full-time salaried employees of the hospital may be able to spend more time with your care than a doctor in private practice, whose income may depend on the number of patients treated. This does not mean that every full-time staff physician will necessarily have generous amounts of time for patient care—their primary responsibilities could be in performing technical procedures, teaching, and research. Nor is it safe to assume that a doctor who is a full-time professor and the head of a department in a teaching hospital will necessarily be a good clinical physician. Professors may be more involved in laboratory research and not be proficient in the clinical management of patients. While a cardiologist's academic or teaching positions may be a helpful guide in establishing his or her credentials, you really need to learn a little more about the physician before making your choice.

In further evaluating the physician, consider the following general guidelines:

Your local public library has a physicians directory, called the *American Medical Directory*, in which all licensed physicians are listed. The directory can answer questions regarding a doctor's schooling, training, certification as a specialist, and memberships in medical associations.

You want a cardiologist who has gone to an established medical school, served a one-year internship and a one- or two-year residency, and done cardiology training. I also recommend that the doctor should be "double-boarded," that is, certified in internal medicine and cardiology. "Board-certified" is a credential granted after passing an examination given by qualified physicians in the specific field. If you learn the doctor is only "board-eligible," it means that the doctor has finished a training program and is considered eligible to take the test. However, the doctor may not yet have taken or passed the examination, or may have failed it one or more times.

Another way to learn whether a cardiologist is board-certified are the initials "FACC," meaning Fellow of American College of Cardiology; the American College of Cardiology is a professional association of cardiologists *who must be board-certified to be full members.* You should not assume that a cardiologist who is not a member of FACC is not board-certified nor is in any way less competent than an FACC member. But certification in the specialty should be a minimum requirement.

As you gather information about possible cardiologists to approach, do not be overly impressed with the reputation of the medical school or university attended. An education at a well-known institution, such as Harvard Medical School, is important, but it does not ensure that the doctor will be an ideal clinician. In fact, the reputation of the hospital the doctor uses or teaches in may be far more revealing. One concern is whether it has medical staff in attendance 24 hours a day. Some private hospitals have a bare staff at night and weekends, or it may have no licensed physicians at all during some of these periods. For example, if you are going to have catheterization, you will want to know whether the hospital has competent surgeons to deal with any emergency situation which may develop. If it doesn't, you might have to endure life-threatening transportation to another hospital.

Finally, your local, state, or national medical association can tell you if any complaints have been lodged against that physician. Incompetency, although rare, may be an issue connected with some physicians.

Personal Recommendation

It should be noted that many physicians direct patients to doctors with whom they have an ongoing professional relationship and from whom they receive reciprocal referrals. I suggest that when you ask for a recommendation from another physician—preferably someone with whom you already have a relationship—ask for the name of a cardiologist to whom this doctor would send a family member, given similar circumstances. Also mention any attitudes or strong feelings (including religious issues) that may affect your care. This approach can be the fastest and perhaps most reliable way to get the best possible referral.

Patient Time

Once you're satisfied you have identified the name of at least one good cardiologist, the next important task is to learn how much time the doctor makes available for patients. Again, you may have to consider the issue of a doctor in private practice versus a full-time hospital staff physician. The doctor in practice may need to see as many patients as possible to sustain the business, possibly as many as one every 10 or 15 minutes. This may be true also of physicians working in a group practice or health maintenance organization (HMO). Another consideration is that at some HMO's you may not always see the same physician on each visit. How many patients the doctor sees in the course of a week or how many hours a week the doctor spends with those patients should be something you can learn without a great deal of trouble. You can ask the doctor's nurse or appointments secretary this type of question. When you call, say quite plainly that you are looking for a cardiologist and you would like to learn how much time the doctor allows for each initial patient visit and follow-up visit, how many patients the doctor sees in a typical week, and how many days or weeks you must wait before the doctor can see you on a nonemergency basis. Also ask how long you should expect to wait in the office, generally, before seeing the doctor? The nurse or secretary may not be able to judge precisely how long each patient must wait, since in the course of the day one emergency can cause disarray to the doctor's entire appointment schedule. You might ask if it's possible to call a few hours in advance of the appointment to learn if there are any major delays.

All this fuss is important because a long wait before seeing your cardiologist, when you may already be worried about your health, can only add to your anxiety. So don't consider these questions of time and schedule impertinent; you're not asking for privileged information. In my view, you should look for someone who can give you forty-five minutes to an hour for your first visit ("the intake"), and at least twenty to thirty minutes for subsequent visits. The number of patients the doctor sees in a week may affect your access: For example, can the doctor usually answer your phone call the same day? Does he or she set aside a fixed time of day to return calls?

Making an appointment with a cardiologist doesn't mean that this doctor must be your permanent choice. I suggest that you make your first visit part of your continuing evaluation. If you decide you and the doctor can work together, do just that. In addition to telling your doctor if something bothers you about your treatment, tell him if something pleases you. He, or she, likes approval, too.

Building Trust

Cardiologists generally expect many of their patients to be anxious, particularly on their first visit. Most patients will have had a cardiac incident or been referred to the cardiologist from another doctor, who has told the patient that he has symptoms of heart disease. Cardiologists also assume that patients will have preconceptions as to what they want in their therapy, whether the ideas are wholly relevant or not. But a good cardiologist wants to hear about them. No matter how foolish you feel, your doctor should be able to explain matters to you and put your fears in perspective.

Some years ago a woman in her middle sixties came to me for treatment of congestive heart failure. She also had a form of leukemia and had been referred to me by her oncologist within the hospital. As soon as she sat down in my office, she told me she did not feel comfortable talking to a doctor young enough to be her son; she preferred an older doctor. At the time, I didn't feel personally rejected. Her concern was expressed as a preference, not an objection. Nevertheless, I sensed that it was a subject she wanted to discuss. I asked her why she had the preference, and she said, "Since I can't reveal anything about my medical problems to my son, why am I going to be able to relate to a doctor his same age?"

Once I asked what it was about her health problem that created this difficulty, she proceeded to relate her fears about her heart disease growing worse and her conviction that her son did not take them seriously. She had been the stalwart figure in her family, providing emotional support especially during times of stress. Now that she was ill, she didn't feel free to divulge the full extent of her illness nor did she believe her son would accept it. Yet at this crucial time in her life, she was the person who needed someone she trusted to take care of her. As we continued to talk, she wept in relief. A sense of trust had already begun to develop between us.

As a result, this woman has become a model patient in that she has not hesitated or delayed, for any reason, to report any development in her health that might require my attention. In addition, we've talked about many other things related to her care, such as different tests, medicines, and diets. But the most meaningful conversations concerned her fear of growing ill and becoming dependent on others. Once she became free of that secret fear, her complicated health picture improved. She now calls me from Palm Beach where she vacations to tell me even when she has a cold. I think she likes to talk about how well she is doing.

Patients whose family members are doctors frequently are treated free of charge as a professional courtesy. This practice can pose a difficulty for some patients: Since they are not paying for the services, they sometimes are reluctant to bother me with "minor" details. An inability to differentiate between "minor" and "major," or a reluctance to call at night in an emergency, can result in inferior care. If you're being seen by any doctor as a professional courtesy, behave as if you were paying for the care. Do not expect a substandard level of care. If for any reason you feel compromised, volunteer to pay as a regular patient.

Another problem can be confidentiality. Last year a patient was referred to me by her husband, another doctor on staff at the hospital. He referred her to me because he had confidence in me as a physician, not because I would treat her free of charge or report back to him everything his wife and I discussed. However, she told me, "I want you to be my doctor, but I can't feel free to tell you everything because I'm afraid that it will get back to my husband." Consequently, the first thing we talked about was the issue of confidentiality. I assured her that anything we discussed in the course of her treatment would not be disclosed to anyone without her permission. I told her that inhibitions can lead to problems in the treatment of heart illness. If you feel you cannot trust your cardiologist, for whatever reason, speak up or find another physician. In the case of patients who are treated as a professional courtesy, I now always ask them directly if they believe not paying for the services will make them less candid or honest with me. It usually clears the air.

One last note on doctor preferences. It is perfectly legitimate to expect that your doctor be someone who does not smoke, is not obese, and generally appears to take good care of his or her personal health. I also think that the doctor's office should reflect care and concern. Is the staff professional and courteous? Does the office have a NO SMOKING sign visibly displayed? While neatness in a doctor's office should not be made a primary requirement, a disheveled-looking office can be disheartening and undermine an early need for confidence.

Your First Visit

Your first visit with your cardiologist, commonly referred to as "the intake," should last from forty-five minutes to an hour. Your doctor's task at this first meeting is to learn enough about you so she or he can treat not the disease but *the patient with the disease.*

The first half of your visit should be devoted to taking your medical history, including some very personal matters. Important questions will concern circulation to other parts of your body: head (strokes, temporary neurological manifestations) and leg (claudication, or cramping, caused by decreased circulation to your legs or muscle cramping when you walk). You should be asked about current medications and should give a detailed history concerning medications you have taken in the past. The doctor will also want you to describe a typical day, the nature of your professional, leisure, and family life, and your family history of illness and allergies. The more information you give the doctor, the greater the likelihood of an accurate diagnosis. If the doctor fails to ask for all the information, give it anyway. If your marriage is stressful, if you drink too much, or if you feel shame about anything that could cause strain on your heart, you risk compromising the quality of your medical care if you don't tell your doctor.

How can you know what information is really important? Thoroughness should be your goal. Specifically, mention the exact symptoms you feel, what precipitated them, what relieved them, and how long you had them. Also, tell your doctor about any prior examination or treatments. You should also share with your doctor any information you fear he will disapprove of, for example, that you are seeing another doctor for the same symptom, or that you are using "recreational" drugs. Remember, all the information you provide about your private life will be held in the strictest confidence.

After getting your personal history, the doctor will examine you physically. One of the first things he'll do is take your blood pressure. A single reading of high pressure presents an incomplete picture of the disease, so it is routine to take several blood pressure readings in both arms during the first visit, especially if the first reading is elevated—above 140/90. I like to take another reading after the patient is rested for a few minutes, since some people have highly *labile* ("not fixed," or "unsteady") blood pressure systems, subject to change depending upon the stress of different circumstances. It's routine to take blood pressure readings during subsequent visits to see if there is a pattern of change in the readings and, of course, to see if a prescribed drug is effective in systematically decreasing high blood pressure. The doctor should do at least a quick examination of your skin, eyes, ears, and mouth for any obvious lesions.

During the intake the doctor will take an extensive history of not only your heart disease but also of all other systems (digestion, breathing, kidney, among others). More time will be expended evaluating your lungs, heart (by listening in several different locations and positions) and the pulses in your neck, arms, legs, and feet.

Cardiac findings can be manifested in unusual ways, even in something as minor as a certain type of fingerprint. A careful examination will reveal such subtle signs and symptoms.

SELF-ASSESSMENT OF
YOUR FIRST VISIT

1. Are you comfortable with the doctor? Did she welcome you warmly?
2. Did you feel rushed during your appointment? Did the doctor listen carefully? Did she grasp all the pertinent information regarding your complaints?
3. Were you encouraged to ask questions and did you understand the answers?
4. Did you mention everything that concerned you?
5. Did the doctor do most of the listening or did she merely take a cursory history and then tell you what you are doing wrong?
6. Did the doctor take notes throughout the entire visit, and did she review her findings or explain her conclusions?
7. Did she conduct a thorough review of your health: gastrointestinal tract, endocrine system, headaches, and joint pains?
8. Did she ask about the medications you are getting?
9. Did she ask about your cardiac risk factor profile: diabetes, hypertension, cigarette smoking, hypercholesterolemia, family history of heart disease?
10. Did she ask when the last time was that you had your cholesterol drawn?
11. Did she ask life-style questions about the sources of stresses and strains in your life, such as work life, married life, sexual history, regular exercise (including whether you drive, ride, or walk to work)?
12. In an emergency, are there doctors who will cover her cases and will these other doctors be familiar with your problems?
13. Did the doctor use analogies to help you understand complex medical problems?

Describing Pain

On your first visit your cardiologist needs to learn what triggers your pains, how often and under what circumstances they occur, and what relieves them. Most important, you need to describe what they feel like. If the doctor leads you to answers by asking you yes/no questions—e.g., "Do you get a sharp pain in your chest?"—it takes away your prerogative to describe the symptoms yourself. Try not to allow yourself to be led to answers the doctor believes are correct. He needs to hear your portrayal of the experience, especially if it concerns coronary pain, more than he needs to have his own suspicions confirmed.

I like to ask my patients this question: "What would you have to do to me in order for me to feel the same discomfort?" Initially some patients are startled by the question, but it usually leads to a more relaxed exchange, sometimes even amusing. One patient told me that he would have to drive a knife into my breastbone; other patients have said they would have to punch me in the chest, or push me. Another said, "Drop a hundred-pound deadweight on your chest." My favorite was the patient who said she would have to drill my teeth.

What's important about this kind of exchange is that pain originating from your heart may not necessarily be classic "chest pressure" radiating to the left shoulder and arm. Because of a complex communication network among the nerves of your body, heart pain may feel like a toothache or a hard tingling in the back, or pain in the jaw, elbow, or stomach. So be prepared to describe the pain in your own language.

Second Opinions and Changing Doctors

Patients change doctors for a variety of reasons. One common reason is to seek a second opinion. Patients often seek another opinion if they are worried about the doctor's recommendation for a particular medical procedure or surgery. I think that second, and even third, opinions are precisely what responsible patients should always consider if they feel they need more advice before making a serious health-care decision. But before speaking to another doctor, I suggest that you try and resolve any conflict or choice you have regarding your care in an open and frank discussion with your original doctor. If the problem can't be resolved, then tell that doctor you are going to ask for another viewpoint so you can feel comfortable with whatever decision is made. You might even ask him or her for a recommendation. You need not use it, but it shows openness and respect for the doctor's professionalism.

When you seek a second opinion from another competent physician, that doctor's viewpoint should also be logical and make sense to you. And merely seeking a second opinion doesn't mean that you must change doctors. In fact, you would benefit most by having the two doctors discuss your problem and come up with a consensus approach.

If you are thoroughly dissatisfied with your doctor's treatment, look for another physician. But far too many people change doctors because they resist a diagnosis they find difficult to accept. Indeed, some people change doctors frequently for this reason. I know of at least two patients who did not want to have surgery, even though four excellent cardiologists recommended it. Hence, these two men continued to change doctors until they found someone who told them that they did not need surgery. In effect, they were treating themselves by looking for a doctor who would agree with their diagnosis. I might add, regrettably, that both men had serious heart attacks within the year.

Choosing Your Surgeon

Most people automatically accept the name of the surgeon who is chosen by their cardiologist. Patients seldom ask questions about the surgeon, thinking perhaps that any questioning would reflect poorly on their cardiologist. Nothing could be further from the truth. It's neither impertinent nor disrespectful to want to learn a few things about someone who will play a very important role in your health care and recovery. Although cardiac surgery is a highly specialized area of medicine, there's no reason you should feel forced to see or accept the surgeon your doctor has recommended. At a minimum, ask your cardiologist to tell you about the surgeon's qualifications and why he or she was chosen. One professional measure of competence I would want to know is how many operations the surgeon performs each year (a minimum of 250), at what hospital, and how many open heart operations does the hospital undertake (a minimum of 500 annually)? Are the surgeon's mortality rates comparable to those of other area hospitals? Does your cardiologist take care of you postoperatively? If the hospital is a community hospital, are physicians available 24 hours in the intensive care unit (ICU) or are the doctors on call from home and nurses take care of emergencies? I would also ask your cardiologist if he or she would be willing to provide the names of one or two other surgeons for you to consider.

TWO

·········

Common Cardiac Illnesses

At this point, I want to talk briefly about how your heart and circulatory system normally works and then describe several heart and cardiovascular diseases that interfere with its normal functions. These descriptions are not meant to be exhaustive—an extended discussion of all coronary heart diseases would be too long and complex for this book. If you want more information about heart disease, consult a more specialized book or your local heart association, an excellent source of teaching material. If you need more information about your own illness, the best source is your cardiologist.

How the Heart Works

Your heart is an organ that's also an astounding muscle, probably the strongest in our body. Probably no other pump, natural or man-made, could equal its performance record. This one-pound organ pumps more than 2,000 gallons of blood each day while beating more than 50,000 times. In effect, our heart pumps three-quarters of a million gallons of blood each year.

The heart, located in the center of your chest behind the breastbone, or sternum, but tilted slightly to the left, is a hollow four-chambered muscular organ consisting of two pumps. When working properly, these pumps rhythmically move blood in and out of your heart as well as throughout some 60,000 miles of blood vessels in your body. The two upper chambers of the heart, called the right and left atria, are separated by valves that act as one-way doors from the two lower chambers, called the right and left ventricles. The right atrium and ventricle, separated by the tricuspid valve, constitute one pump; the left atrium and ventricle, separated by the mitral valve, make up the second pump. There are two other valves: the pulmonary valve controls the flow of blood out of your right ventricle into your lungs, and the aortic valve controls the flow of blood out of the left ventricle into the aorta vessel on its way to the rest of the body. Veins bring blood from the body to the right atrium, and arteries take the blood away from your heart, pumped by the left ventricle, to every single cell in your body. To understand cardiac disease, it is important to understand the normal heart cycle. First, oxygen-poor blood from the veins of your body (the bluish superficial veins seen through your skin) flows into the right atrium and down through the tricuspid valve to the muscular right ventricle. There it is pumped through the pulmonary valve into the lungs, where the carbon dioxide is withdrawn from the red blood cells and fresh oxygen absorbed. From the lungs the blood returns to the heart, where it first flows into the left atrium and then down through the mitral valve into the muscular left ventricle of your heart. There, the oxygen-rich blood is pumped through the aortic valve into the main artery or aorta and delivered to the rest of the body via arteries and finally through tiny capillaries (which give the reddish color to your hands and feet).

Measuring Blood Pressure

Your blood-pressure reading is a measure of the two pressures needed for your heart to function properly, and it is measured at two crucial moments in the heart's cycle: when your ventricles powerfully contract to force blood out of the heart into the aorta, called *systole* ("systolic pressure"); and when the ventricles relax and the mitral valve opens to allow blood to flow back in from the

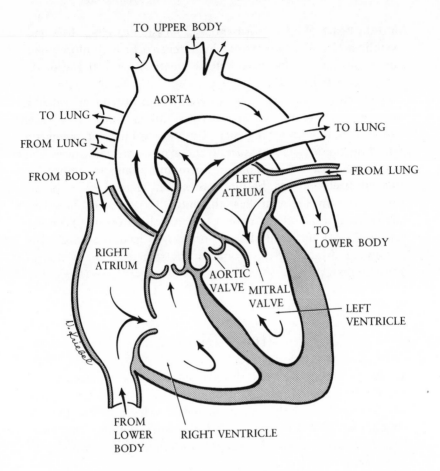

TO UPPER BODY

AORTA

TO LUNG

FROM LUNG

FROM BODY

TO LUNG

FROM LUNG

LEFT
ATRIUM

TO
LOWER BODY

RIGHT
ATRIUM

AORTIC
VALVE MITRAL
VALVE

LEFT
VENTRICLE

FROM
LOWER
BODY

RIGHT VENTRICLE

Roadmap of a Healthy Heart

lungs, called *diastole* ("diastolic pressure"). During these cycles, your diastolic pressure doesn't fall to zero because the aorta maintains a pressure by its elastic properties.

Hence, the higher first number of your blood pressure reading is the high-pressure systolic pumping action needed to drive blood to all the cells of the body. The lower diastolic reading indicates the lower pressure when your heart relaxes to receive the blood back into the heart. While a normal blood pressure can be a 140–100 systolic and a 70–90 diastolic, hypertension or high blood pressure is formally defined as systolic greater than 140 and/or diastolic greater than 90.

Your blood pressure is measured with an instrument called a *sphygmomanometer*, which gives pressure readings on a scale showing millimeters of mercury. The standard measurements are based on the arterial pressure in the arm's brachial artery. The doctor places a cuff around your arm and pumps in enough air to completely cut off the blood pressure. Then she lets the air out slowly, until she can hear the pulse. The pressure shown on the mercury tube at this point is the systolic pressure. Then she lets out more air until she can no longer hear the pulse. The pressure indicated at this point on the mercury tube is the diastolic pressure.

Heart Disease

In this chapter we will discuss specific heart illnesses and symptoms—angina pectoris (from the Latin *angere*, "to choke," and *pectoralis*, "chest") or pain, mitral valve prolapse (MVP), palpitations, hypertension, congestive heart failure, and heart muscle disease—especially in terms of how they are treated with heart drugs.

In general, heart disease can involve the blood vessels, heart valves, or the heart muscle. Cardiac diseases are varied and far too complicated to discuss in great detail here (you can get more detailed information from your doctor). A general description of heart disease is that if for any reason your blood vessels are unable to deliver adequate blood to any muscle, organ, or other tissues of your body, the lack of oxygen can lead to damage, such as a stroke or heart attack. Circulatory diseases develop usually when the blood vessels become too narrow or are blocked, thus restricting the flow of blood-carrying oxygen and other nutrients to the rest of the body. It can be caused by hypertension, high cholesterol, smoking, and diabetes.

Heart Attacks

Coronary circulatory problems occur when the coronary arteries, the blood vessels that carry oxygenated blood directly to the heart muscle, are diseased. When the heart doesn't receive adequate oxygen because of a slowing or blockage of blood flow, a heart attack can occur. An interruption of blood flow can occur in the three major coronary arteries: the left anterior descending (LAD) and the left circumflex (both part of the "left main"), and the right coronary artery. The principle of supply and demand applies: If the supply of fresh blood is adequate for the pumping heart's demands, all is well; however, if the demand increases (for example, during exercise) but the supply is inadequate to meet it, *angina* may develop, which may lead to a heart attack.

Temporary cessation of blood flow (only seconds to minutes) to the heart muscle can cause angina, which is a reversible "cramp" of the heart muscle, while a prolonged cessation of flow will produce a heart attack, or *myocardial infarction*, and perhaps permanent irreversible muscle damage. Interrupted blood flow to the heart tissue may result from a sudden blood clot (*thrombus*) forming in one or more coronary arteries. If a coronary artery goes into spasm, causing a sudden cessation of blood, it can provoke a heart attack.

Coronary Artery Disease

The flow of blood can be slowed by arteries that are narrowed by a buildup of cholesterol. Our blood contains fats, or lipids, necessary for growth and good health, but if we have too much fat in our blood, a condition called *hyperlipidemia*, the excess fat clings to the walls of our arteries and we are at risk of coronary artery disease, or *atherosclerosis*. This buildup of fatty deposits is called *atheroma*. Other major contributing risk factors for coronary artery disease include smoking, diabetes mellitus, a strong family history of coronary artery disease, and hypertension.

As we grow older, the fat buildup along the walls gets thicker and harder and may even calcify, and our blood vessels may become rigid. It is believed that when about three-quarters of a coronary artery is blocked, or *occluded*, the heart muscle may fail to receive enough oxygen during exercise (a condition known as *ischemia*). At 90 percent blockage the supply of blood may be inadequate for even minimal activity, leading to *angina pectoris* (see page 35) or, if prolonged, possibly a heart attack. Once a heart attack occurs, a cascade of events begins which may lead to an irregular heartbeat, or *arrhythmia*, and sudden death.

Spasm

A spasm or convulsive contraction interrupting blood flow in the coronary artery is relatively uncommon but on occasion can cause serious problems; it could cause angina, and might lead to a heart attack. Spasms that last only a few seconds or even minutes might be painful but will not cause any damage. A longer spasm, especially if drug-induced (as with cocaine), that cuts off the flow of blood for five or ten minutes, might permanently harm the heart muscle or even cause a fatal event.

Blood Clot

Your blood is made up of different blood cells circulating in a liquid called plasma. Hemoglobin, the oxygen-carrying component of red blood cells, carries oxygen to all cells in the body; leukocytes, or white blood cells, are needed to defend your body against foreign matter such as bacteria and viruses. Platelets, or thrombocytes, are small, sticky "plugs" that assist in the repair of injured blood vessels by forming clots. (For a further discussion of blood clotting, see page 241.)

The flow of blood is slowed when blood vessels become clogged by a buildup of fat on their walls. Platelets are naturally sticky, and when they pass through the narrowed vessel, they may start to form clots on top of the fat deposits and eventually completely block the flow of blood.

Given enough warning, the body has a strategy to cope with a narrowing blood vessel. A vessel that increases its plaque to

99 percent blockage will close off completely. But to compensate for the progressive narrowing, other neighboring vessels send off branch vessels, or *collaterals*, to the jeopardized muscle. Hence, there may be few symptoms when the vessel closes completely. If a 60 percent lesion (or obstruction) suddenly ruptures and a blood clot completely occludes the vessel, a heart attack will occur. If the blocked artery is in the heart, called *coronary stenosis*, it would cause a heart attack; if in the brain, it might cause a stroke.

If you suffer from high levels of cholesterol in your blood, your doctor will place you on a special diet that restricts your cholesterol and fat intake. If dietary changes are unable to bring blood fat to an acceptable level, your doctor might prescribe drugs that block the absorption of fat into the bloodstream or prevent fat production in the liver. There are two important cholesterol subtypes: *high-density lipoproteins* (HDL), which work to remove fatty deposits from blood vessels, and *low-density lipoproteins* (LDL), which promote plaque progression and fatty deposits. Your goal would be to raise the HDL and lower the LDL (see Cholesterol Screening, page 97).

Indicators of a Heart Attack

Many people fail to recognize the first early signs of a heart attack. Although the most common sign of an injury or a developing disease is pain—this is certainly true of heart disease or a heart attack—the pain of heart disease is not easily recognized as such, in part because the pain of an impending heart attack is not always the same. Patients will frequently say that days or weeks before their heart attack they recall having different kinds of *other* pains that they never thought were related to heart disease. Some patients say that they felt a discomfort high in the stomach or breast bone, which they assumed was indigestion. Another symptom was a pain in the side of the neck, in the jaw, and sometimes a tingling sensation in their teeth, like a toothache. When these symptoms did not grow worse, they thought them harmless and did not think it worth reporting to their doctors, especially if they had not been under the care of cardiologists or had not previously been diagnosed as having heart disease.

What these patients did not realize was that the pain of angina can radiate or travel: It can move to the left shoulder and down the left arm; it can radiate down to your abdomen or up into the small of your back, especially between the shoulder blades or up into the jaw. It also is usually precipitated by some activity or emotional stress. The symptoms these people experienced would not have been dismissed out of hand by a cardiologist, and should not be by any patient with significant heart disease risk factors (see page 88).

People at risk of a coronary attack should be aware of what are called associated symptoms. For example, I know of a man who was anxious about speaking at his grandson's Bar Mitzvah. About an hour before the ceremonies were to begin he developed a gnawing pain in his stomach and burping, which he attributed to overeating the night before. But he grew concerned when he received no relief from Mylanta. Then he realized that the persistent burping and indigestion may be related to his history of angina, although he had never experienced this particular set of symptoms. Ten minutes after he took his nitroglycerin tabs (see page 36), his symptoms disappeared, confirming that they were indeed signs of an anginal attack.

If you have any pain that could be angina, ask yourself whether the pain occurred when you were active or at rest: Indigestion usually isn't brought on by activity, but a cardiac symptom often is. What other circumstances preceded the pain? Have you been under some emotional stress or subject to any other additional pressure during the last week or two?

People in denial about their risk of heart disease often cannot *see* the presence of early signs. The tragedy is that many potential cardiac patients do not take the simple precautions of seeing a doctor for routine checkups for fear of what they might be told. They wait until they have had a significant event, namely, a worsening of their condition or a heart attack. A physician who turned millions of people on to the practice of jogging died from severe coronary disease because he denied that the stomach and chest pains could be cardiac in origin, or that his current rigorously healthful life-style could not erase the prior twenty years of smoking and dietary indiscretion.

Early detection is one of the very best safeguards against a fatal heart attack. If you're at risk for heart disease, pay attention to potential associated symptoms such as unexplained pain or physical signs of discomfort.

If you are alert to the small changes in your health over the years and share those changes with your doctor, you have an opportunity to exercise considerable control over the outcome of your health care. On the other hand, if you resist detection by being inattentive or resist treatment, you are at an increased risk of becoming sick or remaining sick.

Angina Pectoris

The heart muscle receives its needed oxygen from the blood that flows through its three major coronary arteries and their smaller branches. As we have discussed, if the blood supply to your heart briefly becomes insufficient or is blocked (ischemia), it usually causes chest pain or angina pectoris.

Angina pectoris is not a disease but a symptom of one—coronary artery disease. The symptoms of a heart attack, from a tightness, squeezing, or aching in the chest to a sharp pain in the chest, back, arms, or jaw, are essentially similar to angina pectoris, differing primarily in duration. The symptoms are also usually more intense and widespread, and rest or nitroglycerin will not necessarily bring quick relief.

Patients describe the pain of angina in many different ways. Most often it is a tight cramplike grip or a squeezing, crushing feeling that is usually felt in the center of the chest, radiating to the left shoulder and arm and occasionally down to the hand. Others have experienced it as a sharp burning pain often starting in the stomach and spreading to the arms, throat, neck, and jaw or to the middle of the back between the shoulder blades. One elderly patient had new dentures put in, thinking her jaw pain was misaligned dentures. Finally, some patients describe it not as pain but a feeling of heaviness and anxiety or impending doom. Angina may be accompanied by shortness of breath, profuse sweating, nausea, vomiting, palpitations, and fainting.

Angina pectoris may occur during or following strenuous exercise or physical work, intercourse, a heavy meal, walking on a cold and windy day, or periods of intense fear or anger or emotional stress. It can happen at almost any time of the day or night.

The duration of the pain may be only a minute or so; it can also last for ten minutes. A brief seizure or paroxysm of pain suggests that the decreased blood flow to your heart was temporary and probably did little or no damage. However, the longer the pain lasts the greater the risk of some damage to the heart muscle. Angina may be seen as a warning sign that should prompt you to seek medical advice before irreversible damage occurs.

Drugs for Treatment

Angina pectoris is usually relieved by rest and medication, most often nitroglycerin, in the form of a tablet, a spray for under the tongue, or a long-acting patch. Nitroglycerin dilates or opens the normal and blocked arteries, allowing more blood to flow around the blockage to the heart muscle. Two other types of drugs that can reduce not only the pain but the frequency of the angina episodes are beta-adrenergic blockers (see Chapter 7) and calcium channel blockers (see Chapter 8).

Mitral Valve Prolapse (MVP)

The valves of our heart act as one-way doors to allow blood to move into the antegrade or forward chamber and prevent backflow. The valve can malfunction by leaks (*regurgitation*) or by not opening wide enough (*stenosis*). Valve dysfunction can usually be diagnosed by your physician's listening to your heart, and confirmed by an echocardiogram or ultrasound test (see page 107). The two right valves, the pulmonary and tricuspid valves, rarely cause problems. However, disease of the valves on the left, the aorta and mitral valves, can cause severe symptoms. When the opening of the aortic valve narrows from its normal 3 cm to less than 1 cm, called *aortic stenosis*, angina, heart failure, and palpitations can develop. Leakage of the valve, or aorta regurgitation, can cause heart failure and palpitations. *Mitral stenosis* is usually caused by childhood rheumatic fever and can cause palpitations and heart failure, as can *mitral regurgitation.*

Millions of people have a heart valve that fails to close properly, a minor heart abnormality called mitral valve prolapse (MVP). MVP is by far the most common congenital cardiac abnormality and may cause disturbing symptoms, especially in women between the ages of 20 and 40. It occurs in 4 to 5 percent of all women and 2 to 4 percent of all men.

Mitral valve prolapse occurs when the mitral valve does not function properly. In MVP the mitral valve is like a door that is too large for its door frame. When the oxygen-rich blood returns from the lungs and flows into the left atrium, it passes through the mitral valve into the left ventricle, where it's powerfully pumped up through the heart's main blood vessel, the aorta, and out to the rest of the arterial system. However, when the mitral valve closes, as it must so the blood can flow up through the aorta, it may flop or billow backward ("prolapse") into the upper heart chamber or left atrium and may produce a distinctive click heard through a stethoscope. Mitral valve prolapse is also referred to as Barlow's syndrome and click murmur syndrome.

If you have MVP you may have moments of anxiety during the day as you sense some change in your heart rhythm, even an extra beat. In addition to feeling nervous, you may become dizzy, breathless, or a little panicky. Some patients have full-blown "panic attacks" requiring psychiatric intervention. But if your cardiologist has diagnosed the condition properly and feels that it's a minor abnormality, there is no reason for you to think your health is in jeopardy or, worse, that you are in danger of having a heart attack.

In the vast majority of cases, mitral valve prolapse requires very little if any treatment, and it should not restrict you from normal activities. Most important, it does not place you at a higher risk for having a heart attack, although it does place a very small percent of people at a higher risk of other related complications.

Symptoms of MVP

For most people, the only evidence of a mitral valve prolapse is the click or murmur their doctor hears during a routine listening with a stethoscope. However, some people develop periodic palpitations and occasional chest pain. Mitral regurgitation may occur, so that blood may leak back up into the left atrium. On rare occasions, a malfunctioning mitral valve may leak so much that it leads to congestive heart failure.

MVP usually does not require medication, but if the palpitations or fluttery feelings are troublesome, or if the doctor feels an arrhythmia must be corrected, she might prescribe a beta blocker such as Inderal. Another rare complication is the risk of endocarditis, or an infection in the heart (see page 48).

If palpitations or fluttery feelings continue to trouble you, especially if they grow more frequent or increase with exercise, you should tell your doctor. Your physician may want to conduct some tests, such as a 24-hour recording of your heart rhythm (see "Holter monitoring," page 106), to make sure the arrhythmia is benign.

Understandably, MVP patients who complain of chest pains become worried. Many describe the pain as a sharp or sticky feeling that moves down the left side of their chest to their left arm, mimicking anginal pain. Nothing specific may precipitate the pain, although it is most likely associated with periods

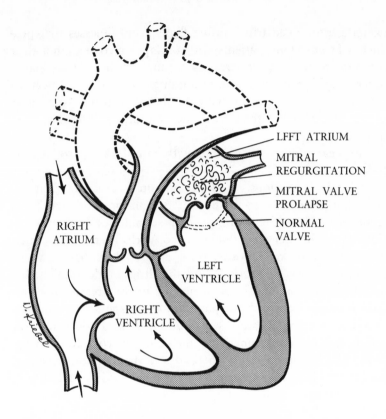

Heart with Mitral Valve Prolapse

of fatigue or stress. I try to assure them that such pains are not evidence of angina or a heart attack, even though they appear similar. The difference is that angina pain gets worse with exercise and eases up with rest or nitroglycerin, whereas chest pain of an MVP is unrelated to strenuous activity. I would urge them to keep a faithful diary (see page 83) and to avoid caffeine, alcohol, stress, and excessive fatigue. I would also check their thyroid gland, for a dysfunction can promote arrhythmia. I also encourage drinking plenty of fluids, particularly following exercise, prolonged trips, airline flights, and illnesses that produce a fever. Many patients with prolapse recognize that their response to anxiety or stress is through their heart, whereas other people react with a fluttering in the stomach or a nervous twitch or blinking. Such patients should confront the cause of the stress rather than treat the resulting palpitations with medicines.

Last year I placed a woman with mitral valve prolapse on Inderal (see page 155) because she had arrhythmia symptoms and was decidedly anxious. A Holter monitor confirmed that the arrhythmia was not serious but the patient was bothered by its recurrence. This drug was especially suitable for her, since besides correcting her arrhythmia it also works on the central nervous system to reduce anxiety. I assured her that although the problem was not serious and the drug would stabilize her heartbeat, the circumstances of her life might occasionally provoke brief episodes of heart palpitations, in spite of the medication, but that she need not worry about them. I added that she should quit smoking, since nicotine could provoke MVP symptoms. The reassurance that she had a fairly common, relatively benign problem was sufficient to relieve her anxiety and most of her symptoms.

Treatment of MVP
Beta-adrenergic drugs such as Inderal are used to treat arrhythmias associated with mitral valve prolapse. If fluid accumulation becomes a complication of heart failure due to MVP, diuretics (see Chapter Six) are used to increase the rate and amount of water and salt the body eliminates, which reduces the amount of fluid the body retains. If atrial fibrillation—a very rapid, irregular arrhythmia—is a problem, your doctor might prescribe digoxin (see page 225), a drug that slows the heartbeat. If you plan to have any dental work done, you should take an antibiotic (see "Endocarditis," page 48) to minimize the very small risk of infection. If the valve function deteriorates, causing severe heart failure, surgery may be required to repair or replace the valve.

Palpitations

The word *palpitations* comes from *palpitatus*, or "throbbing." Clinically, it means the patient is aware of the heart beating, whether it be harder, faster, or with skipped or extra beats. The most common palpitation is when the heart speeds up to work harder to circulate blood to active muscles, such as when exercising. Another common palpitation is the "skipped" beat. Palpitations can suggest a number of different types of problems, but the vast majority of people with arrhythmia or palpitations are not in serious jeopardy of having a heart attack or fainting. In fact, it's not necessary for most of these people to take medication. The primary treatment may be education, reassurance, and life-style changes.

When patients come to me complaining of palpitations, I often ask them to pound out the rhythm of the palpitation on the table. That simple task can be revealing. For example, they might pound out palpitations with a "skip" beat: two light beats, a pause of sorts, and then a heavier beat. Patients are concerned about the missing beat; but they are even more distressed by the fourth beat that is so much more powerful than the others. Once I learn something about the pattern, which may require some tests, I usually can reduce their anxiety by saying that they aren't going to be hospitalized or have a heart attack. Once they learn what the skipped beat means, they are further reassured.

The Missing Beat

A principle of the heart's pumping is that the more the heart fills with blood, the more vigorously it contracts to expel or pump the blood out. An inflated rubber balloon is a good example: Because of its elasticity, the more you fill it with air, the greater the releasing force. In a similar manner, the force with which the heart bounces back is determined by how much it's stretched by the incoming blood. If filled more than is normal, the heart's response will be greater than normal.

When does the heart fill with more blood than is normal? When it has more time for filling. More specifically, if your heart had two seconds instead of one for filling, it will fill more and pump harder.

Let's go back to the patient with the skipped beat. A pulse rate of 60 means one heartbeat per second. At the first second the heart contracts; it contracts again at the next second; but at 2½ seconds, a premature third beat comes in. In effect, the heart fires too soon to contract effectively and a beat is skipped. Consequently, the heart resets its timing, and the next or fourth beat comes on the scheduled fourth second. But because it has an extra half second of filling, the heart contracts with greater force. The skipped beat is called the *compensatory pause*, the pause that causes the greater contraction.

With palpitations, I need to learn the abnormal sequence—different sequences indicate different types of problems—and how frequently someone has the irregular beat and when. Does it happen at certain times of the day? What is the patient doing when it happens? Is it only when he or she is nervous? Is it only at night? One patient admitted that he had been increasing his coffee consumption to almost twenty cups a day because he was in a high-stress job. Once he stopped overstimulating himself with caffeine, the persistent palpitations also stopped.

Once I gather the anecdotal information, and depending upon other clinical data, I might have the patient get an electrocardiogram (see page 104) or place them on a Holter monitor, which is a twenty-four-hour heart rhythm monitor. This device records every single heartbeat and, if an abnormal beat occurs, the time it happened. With the Holter, I will know the total number of irregular heartbeats and their pattern, and any other arrhythmia besides.

If a serious arrhythmia is detected, I might start the patient on a low dose of an antiarrhythmic drug (see Chapter 11). If the situation is more serious, such as a patient with arrhythmia and fainting spells, and the Holter documents that it is a dangerous arrhythmia, I might hospitalize the patient and conduct more tests, and possibly administer an antiarrhythmic drug intravenously. Much can be learned on a Holter. If the arrhythmia is episodic, a small pocket device can catch thirty seconds of a patient's heart rhythm, which can then be transmitted to a nurse-monitored receiving station over the telephone.

But back to our patient with the palpitations. More often than not, patients with palpitations need not be medicated, or if so, for only a limited period. President Bush's arrhythmia was caused by a secondary problem: Graves' disease, or an overactive thyroid gland. One of the symptoms of Graves' disease is rapid or irregular heartbeats. In his case, a simple medication corrected the thyroid gland, which allowed his heart to resume normal functioning, but he needed antiarrhythmic therapy until his overactive thyroid was controlled.

Simply understanding that the palpitations are not life threatening often reduces the patient's anxiety and, hence, the frequency of the palpitations. I usually say something like this: "You're having some extra heartbeats, but none of them are dangerous. Although you may be nervous about them at times, I don't think it is even necessary now for you to take medication. I suggest that you come back in a few weeks and we'll talk about your experience with any palpitations you may have had during that time. Keeping a diary can be very helpful, especially logging in when palpitations occur, their duration, and possible precipitants."

In a few weeks the patients return, usually less troubled and more accepting of their odd condition. Most report very few incidents of irregular heartbeats and they are usually confident that with more changes in their diet and life-style, especially stress reduction, they won't require any further medical attention. They're usually right, too. Some of these patients come to refer to themselves whimsically as people who march to "a different beat." However, persistent and disturbing palpitations always warrant evaluation by your doctor.

Hypertension

Compliance, or following the doctor's orders, is an especially difficult issue with the symptomless disease of hypertension, or high blood pressure. Hypertension's reputation as "the silent killer" is well deserved, since more than twenty-five million people may unknowingly suffer from this disease, and it can be fatal if left untreated. The disease is insidious: it does not occur episodically, but rather progresses steadily, cumulatively, and silently. If unchecked, hypertension's first presentation could be a severe headache, a nosebleed, a stroke, or a heart attack.

Symptoms

Blood pressure is the force that flowing blood exerts against the walls of your blood vessels and organs (see page 29). The action of the heart and the elasticity of the major artery, the aorta, provide the force to drive the blood through the many miles of your arterial system. The proper functioning of the circulatory system depends on three principal factors: a healthy heart, blood vessels that permit a free flow of blood, and a sufficient level of pressure throughout the system to maintain proper blood flow.

Higher levels of pressure are caused by an increased resistance to blood flow. Usually, the increased resistance results because the passageways in your blood vessels have become too narrow, and this can happen when the muscles in the vessel walls, which are influenced by the autonomic and central nervous systems and the hormonal system, become more constricted, reducing the room for blood to flow. Faced with the increased resistance, the heart must work harder, i.e., increase the force at which it pumps every single beat (60 to 80 times a minute), every minute of every hour of every day. And, like any other muscle that gets a vigorous and steady workout, the heart muscle grows thicker and stiffer. The excessive levels of pressure continually exerted on the walls of your blood vessels and organs gradually cause damage.

When explaining to my patients what it's like for the heart to

44

labor under the demands of hypertension, I ask that they imagine a faucet. Like a faucet turned on and off rhythmically, your heart rhythmically exerts steady pressure to produce a gentle surge of blood. Faced with increased resistance of high pressure in the blood vessels, the heart must be "turned on" sharply, producing a blood flow that is harsh and rapid. The "turn on" is the systolic pressure. The hydrostatic pressure in the pipes that maintains pressure so the water is ready to flow immediately is diastolic. If the faucet is partially clogged, you have to turn the faucet hard to generate flow: With increased resistance your heart has to pump harder.

A persistent level of elevated blood pressure adversely affects more than just your heart; it can cause damage to all your organ systems, especially your eyes, brain, and kidneys. Hypertension can cause the small capillaries of the eyes to hemorrhage and impair vision; it can rupture the blood vessels in the brain and produce a stroke; it can be life threatening if it blocks blood flow to the kidneys; and if it damages the blood vessels of the heart, it can cause a heart attack.

Its lack of symptoms makes early detection of hypertension difficult. Because the disease is "silent," you will not be aware of the hypertension until you have your blood pressure read, during a routine physical check-up or when you give blood. Another less fortunate time may be when something serious goes wrong.

Treatment of Hypertension

The treatment of hypertension has changed in recent years: new drugs and a greater reliance on nonpharmacologic treatments such as weight loss, low-salt diets, and reduced alcohol consumption are routine.

In the case of very mild hypertension, your doctor may first recommend you lose any excessive weight, restrict your salt intake, and, where appropriate, make changes in your daily routine that could reduce stress. If these strategies are not successful, your doctor may include medication as part of the treatment. If your hypertension is severe, she may start you on drugs immediately.

Hypertension can range from mild to life threatening, and patients also may respond differently to a particular treatment. Consequently, different approaches have been recommended for the treatment of hypertension. The American Heart Association and the Joint National Committee on Detection, Evaluation and Treatment of High Blood Pressure have recommended that a progressive, or stepped, approach be used in the management of this disease.

Generally, Step 1 involves the use of a single drug, most often a diuretic or beta blocker, combined with nonpharmacological treatments. Diuretics increase the rate and amount of water and salt the body eliminates, thereby reducing high pressure. The other category of drugs are beta blockers. By blocking the effects of the stimulant epinephrine, the drug causes the heart to beat more slowly and less forcefully. Your doctor will properly prescribe relatively low doses initially, unless your hypertension is considered dangerously high.

If Step 1 is not effective in controlling your high blood pressure, your doctor will move to Step 2 and prescribe both a diuretic and a beta blocker, and possibly add a third drug. Depending upon the effectiveness of this step, your doctor may add a vasodilator-type drug, which works by dilating the arteries, reducing resistance to blood flow and thus the heart's work load. In some instances, patients may be taking four separate drugs to both treat their blood pressure and reduce the potential for side effects of one or more of the drugs.

Two other types of drugs, calcium channel blockers (see Chapter 8) and angiotensin-converting enzyme (ACE) inhibitors (see Chapter 9) help reduce high blood pressure by dilating the narrowed arteries and increasing blood flow.

Congestive Heart Failure

Congestive heart failure (CHF) means that the heart pumps inefficiently, reducing the flow of blood flow to the muscles, tissues and organs of the body. If the pumping action becomes very weak, blood may back up behind the heart and fluid may accumulate in the tissue around the lungs or in other body tissue. Symptoms include edema, or a swelling of the legs or ankles, and difficult breathing. Pulmonary edema is an extreme condition in which the lungs are virtually drowning in fluid, causing severe shortness of breath.

Congestive heart failure occurs for a variety of reasons: muscle damage following a heart attack, valve dysfunction, primary muscle disease, or hypertension. It's always considered a serious condition that can become life-threatening.

Symptoms of CHF

The symptoms of congestive heart failure are usually progressive. Initially, patients feel weak and tire easily. They also become breathless, first after exercise and then during normal work routines. It's possible that trouble breathing will occur only when you lie down to go to sleep at night. Another symptom of congestive heart failure is edema or a swelling in the ankles and feet. Some patients will also have swollen neck veins and an enlarged liver. If the disease has progressed, the patient may have an enlarged heart or congested lungs, too.

Treatment of CHF

In addition to plenty of rest and a low-salt diet, diuretics are commonly used to treat CHF to increase the rate and amount of water and salt the body eliminates; this reduces both the swelling in the legs and the fluid in the lungs that causes the breathlessness. Digitalis preparations can also be effective, as they cause the heart to beat more forcefully and can correct certain heart arrhythmias as well. Vasodilators and beta blockers may also be recommended to reduce arrhythmias.

Heart Muscle Disease

When some part of the heart muscle is structurally damaged or defective, but no cause is found, it's called a *cardiomyopathy*.

Cardiomyopathies occur in a variety of circumstances: If the heart is dilated and thin-walled, and it cannot effectively pump blood (*dilated congestive cardiomyopathy*); if the heart chambers become thick and enlarged, or if the walls of the left ventricle become so thick and stiff, they actually obstruct the blood exiting the heart (*hypertrophic cardiomyopathy*); if the general heart muscle stiffens so it cannot expand and fill with blood (*restrictive cardiomyopathy*).

Symptoms

Often there are few if any symptoms of cardiomyopathy until the disease is in an advanced state. The symptoms may range from breathlessness, fainting spells, and edema to heart palpitations and chest pain. In other instances, the first sign of the disease is a heart attack.

Treatment

Treatment for cardiomyopathy depends upon the type of disease and severity of the symptoms. In the most severe cases, a heart transplant may be necessary. But if the damage is less serious, diuretics can reduce the symptoms of edema, beta-adrenergic blockers and calcium channel blockers can relax the stiff muscle, and vasodilators and digitalis drugs can help improve cardiac output. Treatment for the cardiomyopathy with weak heart muscle includes rest, vasodilators, and avoidance of heavy physical exertion.

Endocarditis

People with certain heart conditions are at risk for developing an infection in the heart itself. Endocarditis (*endocardia* means "within the heart") is an infection of the lining or the valves of the heart. It rarely occurs in people with normal hearts; the people at an increased risk—although still a statistically small percentage of the population—are those who have damaged heart valves from heart disease such as mitral valve prolapse, rheumatic fever, or a congenital defect. People with artificial heart valves or who have a history of bacterial endocarditis are at even greater risk.

The infection develops when bacteria gets attached to an abnormal heart valve, or heart tissue that has been damaged. Once lodged, the bacteria produces a growth that can eventually damage or destroy the valve. The growth can also break off, move through the bloodstream, and block an artery, a condition called an *embolus*. A blocked artery is very serious: In the brain, a blocked artery can produce a stroke; in a coronary artery it can cause a heart attack.

Symptoms

One quite rare form of this disease, acute endocarditis, can develop rapidly even on normal heart valves, causing high spiking fevers, chills, and heart murmurs. If untreated it can be fatal within days or weeks.

The onset of subacute endocarditis, both on previously damaged and normal heart valves, is usually more gradual, but its symptoms are more insidious, masquerading as weight loss, low-grade fever, anemia, malaise, and chronic fatigue syndrome. This form of endocarditis responds better to treatment than acute endocarditis.

Many patients with endocarditis develop a low-grade fever and feel an achiness in their muscles. They may also experience some chest pain and unexplained weight loss.

Treatment

Treatment for endocarditis depends upon the nature of the infectious agent (type of bacteria or fungus) and the severity of the symptoms. Generally intravenous antibiotics are given for several weeks, until well after symptoms have disappeared, to ensure that all the bacteria have been eliminated. If the heart failure continues, fevers or an emboli may develop. Surgical removal and replacement of the infected valve might be warranted. The disease could cause abscesses to develop on the heart, which would have to be drained.

Prevention

Bacteria get into your blood in a variety of ways. Most commonly, bacteria form in your mouth or in a wound. Usually the bacteria are destroyed quickly before they can do any damage. However, it pays to keep your teeth well brushed and flossed. Dental procedures that cause bleeding, whether a simple cleaning, filling a cavity, or a surgical procedure, increase the risk of bacteria reaching your bloodstream. In these circumstances endocarditis can occur, primarily in people with abnormal heart valves unless, of course, they have taken antibiotics to combat the bacteria.

If you are at risk for endocarditis and you plan to have dental work done, make sure you receive two doses of an antibiotic, preferably Amoxicillin: one dose of 3 grams orally at least an hour before the procedure and a second dose of 1.5 grams about six hours after the first dose. If you are allergic to Amoxicillin or penicillin, your dentist should give you erythromycin ethylsuccinate or stearate erythromycin. (If you were in a hospital undergoing surgery for the gastrointestinal or genitourinary tract, you would probably receive an intravenous or intramuscular antibiotic.)

One worried patient actually told me she had considered designing for herself a daily regimen of antibiotics to prevent any such infection from occurring. She desisted when I told her that she is at risk only when dental work is done, or during any kind of surgery. Besides, regular use of an antibiotic would likely lead to bacteria developing a resistance to the drug, which could leave the woman more vulnerable to infection.

THREE

....

Medications

Between 1968 and 1988 the death rate due to coronary heart disease (CHD) plunged 48 percent. Millions of lives were saved and others greatly extended by developments in heart disease treatment, principally the effective use of new surgical procedures and, perhaps more important, new drug regimens.

Heart drugs affect the lives of virtually all heart patients; some take medications temporarily, while others take them for the remainder of their lives. But as millions of people begin to take some form of cardiovascular drugs each year, many do so without sufficient understanding of what the drugs do.

What Heart Drugs Can—
and Cannot—Do

Heart drugs do not *cure* heart disease. Drugs usually are able to reverse the symptoms but not reverse the existing damage. For example, a heart drug designed to treat coronary artery disease may reduce the work of the heart so the body needs less blood, in effect, helping the heart and body to accommodate themselves to the new situation. Other heart drugs may reduce the likelihood of the disease, for example blood clot formation, growing worse or recurring.

Angina medications provide an example of how heart drugs can allay symptoms. Angina is caused by a decreased blood supply to specific regions of the heart muscle, usually because a blood vessel is partially blocked. Nitrates work to dilate the vessel to increase blood flow, and beta blockers and calcium channel blockers slow the heart rate and force of contraction, and decrease energy demands on the heart. In neither instance do the medications reverse the disease process; they only counteract its effects. The underlying blockage will remain and may progress, despite a patient's religious adherence to a drug regimen.

Drugs taken for essential hypertension—the most common form of hypertension and for which there is no known cause—provide another example. Although hypertensive drugs cannot correct or cure the underlying mechanisms that cause essential hypertension, they nevertheless can effectively reduce or eliminate the symptoms, which may allow your body to recover to almost normal functioning. Diuretics can reverse the tension on the blood vessels by drawing excess water from the tissue surrounding them, which relaxes the pressure on the vessel walls and thus eases the work of the heart. Antiarrhythmic drugs can suppress the irregular electrical firing in the heart and correct heart palpitations, but they cannot alter the primary cause that produced the arrhythmia in the first place. Of course, if the arrhythmia is the result of a secondary problem, such as hyperactive thyroid, then the drug designed to correct the thyroid function can be said to "cure" the arrhythmia as well.

There is one type of antihypertensive drug that seems to reverse the disease process: calcium antagonists. Hypertension can cause the heart muscle to thicken, which predisposes the patient to a heart attack. When calcium antagonists are used to bring blood pressure within a normal range, the drug can actually reverse the thickening of the heart muscle, which then returns to normal size. Lipid-lowering drugs are also believed to be curative—when used in conjunction with a low-cholesterol diet, they may actually cause regression of blood vessel plaque.

Drugs of the future offer great promise. It is thought that certain drugs will not only suppress the symptoms of heart disease, but will probably prevent the physiological changes that lead to certain forms of heart disease, such as high blood pressure. Studies of the function of receptor sites, the parts of the cell that control the thousands of different actions in the body, have led researchers to believe that defects in these receptors are the cause of most heart disease. It's also believed that drugs will be able to correct these defects and greatly reduce the incidence of heart disease in the near future.

The heart drugs available today, however, do not cure heart disease; they only subdue or eliminate the symptoms. Still, if we take the time to learn what our heart drugs are capable of doing and how to take them properly, they will help us to lead virtually normal lives.

One of the most common questions about heart drugs I hear is "Will I have to take this drug the rest of my life?" Sometimes my answer will be yes, but more often it is no, or at least "not as much and not as frequently." Regardless of the drug, however, daily or seasonal variations in your need for the drug will be evident over time. As you get older your disorder will need reevaluation periodically. So even if you have been told that you'll probably have to take a drug for the remainder of your life, advances in medicine could change this prediction or might make it more convenient for you in the future.

Changing Drug Schedules

It's important that you ask your doctor at various periods whether the use of a particular drug can be reevaluated. If you're being treated for high blood pressure, you should have your doctor consider reexamining the details of your drug treatment as soon as your pressure has been normal for at least a year. At that time he should look to reducing the dosage of your antihypertensive medication while you make renewed efforts to explore nonpharmacological strategies, such as relaxation techniques and dietary regimens. Such a review is especially important if you have had to take a number of heart medications for a year or more. At some point your doctor should be able to eliminate one or more of the drugs, or at a minimum reduce the dosage of one or all drugs. Even if you were taking only one heart drug, the dosage might still be reduced, or it could be exchanged for another more convenient medication that's easier to take. A review would also be considered appropriate after several months if you were taking certain medications following a heart attack or open-heart surgery.

With almost any drug regimen, your doctor will initially prescribe one or more medications and watch how you and your disease respond to them, especially regarding any potential side effects, adverse reactions, specific tolerances and allergies, and variations in metabolic rates. On the basis of his observations he may make adjustments in the drug regimen to meet your unique needs. This monitoring procedure is important, as no two people necessarily respond the same way to a specific drug, nor will one person always respond to the same drug in the same manner. Changes in our constitutional health, metabolism, or emotional disposition, environmental influences, and other sensitivities affect our response to a medication. With extended use, we may also develop a tolerance toward the drug that could reduce its effectiveness and necessitate a change.

Although changes are the rule, I always expect my patients to follow my directions concerning the use of their medications. Strictly following the schedule, however, means more than just taking them on time. It also means you don't, for whatever reason, discontinue the drug, change the dosage or brand of drug, or take someone else's medication without your doctor's knowledge.

Sharing Drug Information

Patients of mine routinely speak to their friends about details of their treatment; it can be comforting for them, but also confusing.

Two patients who have had open-heart surgery may not necessarily have similar subsequent therapies. The drug treatment following open-heart surgery for severe coronary disease will differ from the treatment after surgery for valve replacement. And even if two people were both to have valve surgery and similar scars on their chests, one may have had repair of a heart valve, while the other may have had surgery to replace a valve with a metal valve— each requiring different drug therapies. Patients with valve-repair surgery may need very few medicines for a limited period of time, while those with metal valve replacements may need to take anticoagulants for the rest of their lives. Hence, open heart surgery patients often have unique postoperative drug treatments.

I recall a heart patient telling me that while at church one Sunday, he complained to a friend of a mild chest discomfort and a burning feeling in his stomach. His friend, a fellow heart patient, innocently diagnosed it as angina and gave him one of the small nitroglycerin tablets he carried. My patient immediately felt faint and had to be taken to an emergency room. While probably well meant, his friend's advice was dangerous: first, the patient's symptoms proved to be indigestion, not angina; second, even a tiny amount of nitroglycerin can be dangerous if taken without a proper diagnosis and supervision.

Another example is people who believe that diuretics are basically the same. Diuretics are not the same: one might be long-acting and the other not; or one may contain a powerful antihypertensive drug while another may be designed specifically to spare potassium. Exchanging heart drugs of any type can cause major problems and may in some instances be lethal.

A lovely 65-year-old woman patient calls me periodically about her mild hypertension, always following an afternoon playing bridge with her friends, because in addition to playing cards they compare diseases and treatments. Usually, I have to explain that while she and her friend may both have coronary disease, the other woman may not have high cholesterol or a hyperactive thyroid as she does. Moreover, if her friend has a history of kidney disease, it would call for a slightly different dosage or drug.

This issue of sharing drugs may be even more important in light of a recent trend of drug companies to appeal to the public through television and newspaper ads. Although the public cannot purchase these prescription drugs on their own, they can ask or even pressure their doctor about their use. One widely publicized survey described "alarming" changes in blood cholesterol and glucose metabolism as a result of a particular diuretic. The story received widespread publicity and appeared in more than 200 newspapers and television stories. It also caused tens of thousands of patients to express their concerns to their doctor regarding the reported side effects of the drug, even though their hypertension had been successfully controlled for years by their diuretic therapy. This attempt to market prescription drugs directly to consumers is a great concern to physicians because we fear that it might wrongly lead some patients to greater unsupervised use of their drugs.

How Heart Drugs Work

Different heart drugs have different actions. Certain drugs, for example beta blockers, act on a part of the cell called a receptor. Other drugs, such as digoxin, affect the chemical composition within cells: Digoxin increases intracellular calcium, which is needed for a more forceful contraction; antiarrhythmics work on the sodium and potassium concentration within cells to affect electrical conduction and excitation. The effectiveness of a drug may be a function of how it is metabolized, how fast it is broken down and thus how long it remains effective. Knowing more about how some of these drugs work may help you better understand how they can help you.

Drug Metabolism
Some part of everything you eat or consume is metabolized, that is, broken down and prepared for absorption. The process begins

with your saliva upon swallowing and continues in your stomach and intestines. Food is broken down and absorbed into your bloodstream and transported to the body. Anything that is not metabolized is excreted without being absorbed into your bloodstream.

The same is true of drugs. After you take a drug, its therapeutic components are absorbed into your bloodstream and the by-products that are not absorbed are eliminated in your urine. Certain drugs become activated only after they are metabolized because the by-product of their metabolization process, the *metabolite*, is the active drug.

Most medicines are absorbed and circulated throughout the entire body system, which means that heart drugs will affect systems other than your heart such as your stomach and brain. The extent of these other effects in large measure determines whether a drug is prescribed or discontinued.

Some people metabolize and absorb their foods more quickly and efficiently than others. Some people have difficulty absorbing fats, while others absorb the mineral iron or specific vitamins poorly. In the same manner, drug metabolic rates differ from person to person.

The rate at which we break down and absorb a drug is influenced by a number of factors. The time it takes for some drugs to reach our bloodstream is determined by the presence of food, other drugs, our age and general health, and how active we are. People who are highly active or have a fever will have an increased metabolic rate. As a group, the elderly metabolize their drugs more slowly. Foods can influence absorption; for example, tea may decrease iron absorption. These factors can cause our metabolic rates to change on a day-to-day basis.

Drug Tolerance

A major innovation in dispensing certain drug medications has been the "patch," which is stuck like a Band-Aid on the skin to deliver a steady amount of a drug over a long period of time. Patches are used to administer scopolamine to people with motion sickness and may in the future be used for birth control drugs. In cardiology, patches are used to deliver a steady amount of nitro-glycerin to patients with angina. The patch is a wonderful innovation because it is convenient and reduces noncompliance in many patients. But patients can also develop drug tolerance with the use of nitrate patches.

If the receptor is constantly bombarded with the drug, at some point it will no longer respond and the effectiveness of the drug will cease. With nitroglycerin patches, when it was recommended that patients remove the patch before going to bed and put on a new one in the morning, their anginal pain disappeared. Removing the patch at night before going to bed gave the receptor a necessary respite from the drug, making it more effective.

Many drugs require a specific interval between doses to allow blood levels to come down, yet stay within the range in which the drug remains effective. An example is Isordil. Initially, cardiologists prescribed Isordil every four hours for the treatment of angina. But it became clear that the longer a patient took the drug the less effective it became: Our patients were developing a tolerance. Prescribed at a four-hour frequency, it saturated the receptors, but at intervals of six to eight hours, the drug maintained its effectiveness and tolerance was no longer an issue for most patients.

Receptor Sites

A receptor is a component of the cell that, when stimulated, alters the function of the cell. Without receptors our bodies could not function. We could not respond to stimuli outside our bodies, such as sight, hearing, or touch; other receptors are designed to respond to internal stimuli, such as the influence of hormones. Receptors are also classified on the basis of what stimuli they respond to, such as light or pressure or chemicals. The receptors that concern us are those affected by specific hormones our body produces and specific heart drugs.

Heart drugs work on a number of receptor sites, but primarily those that affect the heart and blood vessels. The relationship between receptor sites and drugs can be likened to an electrical socket and plug: the socket is the receptor and the medication is usually the plug. Inotropic drugs are drugs designed to stimulate the receptor site of the heart muscle when the heart requires more force to pump. Some heart drugs act to block the receptor site, in effect barring the body's natural stimulants from reaching the socket. For example, some beta blockers block receptor sites so that the hormone epinephrine, a normal stimulant of the heart, cannot reach the cell and stimulate the heart muscle. This is important if the heart needs to beat less rapidly.

Certain beta-blocker medications are "receptor-specific," that is, they affect only B1 receptors on the heart, whereas other beta blockers influence those sites plus others. B1-selective beta-adrenergic blockers (e.g., Lopressor and Tenormin) affect just the cardiac or heart (B1) receptors, whereas nonselective beta-adrenergic blockers (e.g., Inderal and Blocadren) also affect the B2 receptors, which are located in the lungs and blood vessels. The nonselective beta blockers might precipitate asthma and other breathing problems in people with a susceptibility toward those problems. These heart patients can take the B1-selective beta blockers since these drugs will have fewer, if any, side effects on the lungs.

Blood Levels

The goal of drug therapy is to provide and maintain an appropriate effective amount of the drug in our blood. Because the drugs we consume are metabolized over one period of time and used by the body over another, the amount in our blood will vary, or rise and fall, during the interval between scheduled doses.

Let us assume that the therapeutic or ideal blood level for a particular drug is 4 particles per thousand. If blood levels reached 8 particles per thousand, it would be toxic and dangerous; if it fell below 2 parts, it would be ineffective. The blood level at which the drug would be most effective in eliminating symptoms of the disease, the drug's *therapeutic window*, would be levels between 2 and 7 parts per thousand.

If you were to take this medication at eight o'clock in the morning, it might take about an hour for the level to reach 2 particles per thousand. Over the next four to six hours, the level might rise to about 6 parts, and then come down to around 2 parts for the last two hours or so. About that time, you should take the next dose. That's ideal.

Although this drug may be prescribed every six hours, you might discover that you consistently metabolize it faster than what was typical or expected: Your blood levels might fall below 2 parts per thousand before you were to take your next dose—and your symptoms might regularly recur as a result.

Over a period of weeks or months, you might discover that you metabolize your medication differently from day to day, depending upon your diet and activity level. Here again, you would learn that your blood level has fallen to a point below our example of 2 parts per thousand only when your symptoms returned.

How do you learn if you are metabolizing your drug faster than anticipated? One sign, of course, is a recurrence of your symptoms, probably just before your next scheduled dose. But telling your doctor that you get symptoms several hours after you take your medication is not very precise. Your doctor would also want to learn how many times the symptoms recur, at what intervals or how far apart, and what you were doing at those moments. Our memories can be very imperfect, especially when discussing a serious illness in our doctor's office.

Levels of certain medications can be measured by a routine blood sample. However, if you keep an accurate and precise diary that records when you took the drug and when you have symptoms and what relieves them, you and your doctor might see a pattern unfolding. Consulting such a record, your doctor would see with greater accuracy what the problem was and alter your therapy accordingly. From studying your own records you might also gain some welcome assurance before your next doctor's visit that your symptoms probably did not mean that your disease was getting worse, but only that your medication needed adjustment.

In our example of a rapid metabolic rate, your doctor might make one of two adjustments to prevent your medication level from falling below therapeutic levels: prescribe a larger dosage each time, or have you take the medication every four hours instead of every six. The individualizing of your medication, or *titration*, is an ongoing process.

Last year, a woman in her twenties came to me with mitral valve prolapse (see page 36). Generally it is not a serious problem and does not make a person sick. This woman was slim, energetic, and an avid swimmer. She took the medication faithfully every eight hours as prescribed. After about three weeks, however, she discovered that her heart would occasionally race. She was worried that her condition was growing worse and called me. I asked her to come in so I could examine her and look at the diary she was keeping. There we discovered that the palpitations occurred about two or three times a week, and always late in the day or about six hours after she had taken her Inderal. She had not quit smoking, either.

I explained to her that although the drug was intended to last eight to twelve hours, it might not. I was sure she was metabolizing the drug faster than the norm, since active people in their twenties will more rapidly metabolize drugs than people in their fifties. A change to a six-hour interval seemed to correct the problem. Once the adjustment was made, she seldom experienced any palpitations and her confidence in the medication grew. The reduced incidence of palpitations may also have been tied to the fact that she successfully quit smoking.

Another alternative might have been to prescribe a long-acting preparation, which remains in the bloodstream for a long period of time. However, sometimes a long-acting preparation is ineffective, since patients can develop tolerance to them. I generally prefer *initiating* therapy with a shorter-acting drug to ascertain the patient's response, to both the drug's intended effect and its side effects, since a longer-acting drug can produce longer and more persistent side effects.

Discontinuation or Withdrawal

A decision to stop taking your medications because you are feeling better may have catastrophic ramifications. If certain drugs are stopped abruptly, they can produce a *rebound effect*, where the original symptoms of the illness recur. If the receptor site that had been blocked suddenly has full access to a stimulant, it may become overwhelmed or overstimulated. If beta blockers, for example, are not slowly tapered, so the receptor site is permitted to grow accustomed to the body's natural stimulation, you may well have angina pain again. Sometimes, the rebound pain is intense. Hence, whenever you are going to discontinue the use of a hypertensive medication, be sure to do it slowly and taper off the use of the drug over a number of days. You should be under a physician's guidance whenever you begin to take a drug or discontinue one.

Multiple Drug Schedules

The treatment of heart disease frequently involves more than treating a single illness with a single drug. More than half of all patients being treated for cardiac illnesses take more than one drug and many are being treated for more than one disease. Some patients may take three or more drugs. As a result, patients who are taking different types of medications need to be especially disciplined about following their doctor's instructions as to how and when to take them. If you are taking drugs prescribed by a doctor other than your cardiologist, it's important to let your cardiologist know what they are, the dosages prescribed, and how often you are supposed to take them.

Whether taken simultaneously, the same day, or even the same week, specific combinations of drugs can adversely increase or decrease each other's effectiveness to the point that one or more of the drugs may become either ineffective or highly toxic.

My advice is to bring a sample of all the drugs you are taking with you on your first office visit. Once your cardiologist knows what medications you're taking, he can create an integrated regimen. I frequently give the patient an index card with one pill of each medication pasted on it with directions for taking it. This card is a reminder for the patient and is brought to each visit so any changes in the drug regimen can be made on it.

If your doctor is not aware of all the medications you are taking, you may be placing yourself at risk of an adverse reaction. For example, a heavily promoted prescription antihistamine, Seldane (terfenadine), can affect your electrocardiogram reading and, in rare instances, produce arrhythmia.

Another example: one of my patients with congestive heart failure was also being treated for a gastrointestinal disorder. Her gastroenterologist had prescribed Tagamet, a drug that can inhibit the absorption of other drugs. She did not tell me she was taking Tagamet, so I could not understand why the drug I was prescribing was so significantly ineffective after more than two weeks of use. Once I learned about the Tagamet, we changed to a new drug that was not adversely affected by Tagamet. Almost immediately she responded better.

Far more common are patients who fail to tell me they are treating themselves for allergy or common cold symptoms. I suppose such problems are so commonplace that it does not occur to them to tell their doctors. But medicines that are used to treat allergy or cold symptoms often contain an antihistamine, which can slow the heartbeat. Bronchodilator-decongestants used to treat cold symptoms contain a pseudoephedrine-type medication whose effect is to stimulate the heart. Depending upon the nature of your heart disease and the drugs you are taking, a bronchodilator or an antihistamine could cause serious problems when taken with various heart drugs.

What is even more commonly unreported by my patients is the use of antacids, because no prescription is needed and they are not thought of as medicine. Yet antacids can easily inhibit the absorption of many heart drugs. If your doctor doesn't realize you have been taking antacids, he may unnecessarily and dangerously increase the dosage of your heart medication. The danger in this situation is that the higher dosage can easily produce an adverse reaction; also, should you stop use of the antacid you might quickly begin to absorb far more of the heart drug than was needed and develop a toxic response.

Aspirin, probably our most commonly used drug—though most patients don't view it as a drug—has significant ramifications. Aspirin reduces the effects of platelets to form blood clots, whether in broken blood vessels on the skin or internally. Also, it can dangerously increase the effect of anticoagulants, such as Coumadin. Coumadin and aspirin would never be prescribed together, as they are contraindicated. However, many people take the two drugs together, often unwittingly and sometimes with disastrous results.

As a nonnarcotic analgesic that relieves pain and reduces inflammation and fever, aspirin has been available since 1899. This remarkably popular drug also acts as an antiplatelet agent in the prevention of blood clots. Many of my patients ask about the benefit of taking one aspirin a day to prevent blood clots.

In a recent Harvard physicians' study conducted to determine what is the best treatment to prevent blood clots, aspirin was one of the drugs that proved to reduce the incidence of heart attacks and strokes caused by blood clots. The research also revealed that, contrary to popular opinion and practice, daily aspirin use was not a totally safe prophylactic. In fact, in that study an aspirin a day appeared to increase the incidence of intracerebral bleeding. It was concluded that people without any risk factors of heart disease or evidence of cerebral circulation problems should *not* take aspirin on a daily basis.

When you're taking an anticoagulant, always discuss it with your doctor before taking any other medicine. The regular use of aspirin can increase the anticoagulating potential of Coumadin, or any other anticoagulant, and cause excessive bleeding. Since people are unaware that many OTC preparations contain aspirin, patients often unwittingly consume aspirin-containing products (e.g., Midol and Alka-Seltzer) while taking an anticoagulant and create mild to serious bleeding problems. Hence, it's important to check the labels of OTC products, such as cough capsules and hay fever products, before using them. Other analgesic products, such as indomethacin and ibuprofen—sold as Indocin, Nuprin, or Motrin—can also result in adverse interactions with anticoagulants.

Beta blockers are safe and effective cardiovascular drugs for most patients. But for those who suffer from diabetes or asthma, these relatively safe drugs can cause serious problems. If you have a significant fluctuation of blood sugar or a history of asthma, even if you have not had any symptoms or an attack for years, certain types of beta blockers should not be given to you (see page 59).

Although different drugs can be taken safely together, what's unsafe is when your doctor does not know all the drugs you are taking.

WHEN A HEART DRUG IS PRESCRIBED

When your doctor prescribes a medication, you should ask for the following information:

1. Why has the drug been prescribed?
2. Will it affect my life-style, such as exercise or drinking alcohol?
3. What are its more serious potential side effects or adverse reactions? Will it affect my sex drive or level of concentration?
4. What do I do if I have any specific side effects?
5. Will it interact with any other drugs, including over-the-counter (OTC) medications?
6. Should the drug be taken with or without food? Must I avoid any specific food, alcohol, or vitamins while taking the drug? If so, why?
7. When should drugs be taken and how much? Should they be taken all at the same time?
8. How should I alter my medication regimen if I must fast for a day for religious reasons?
9. How soon will the drug take effect?
10. How long will one pill be effective?
11. How long will I take the drug (the "trial period") before the dose will be adjusted?
12. Do I need to wake up at night to take the drug or take it only when I am awake? ("Three times a day" usually means while you are awake, whereas "every eight hours" means around the clock).
13. What do I do if I miss my scheduled dose? Should I take it immediately, take it with the next dose, or skip it altogether?
14. If the capsule is too large, and I am not permitted to chew it, can I mix it with water or juice or soft foods?
15. Are there any special precautions for pregnant or nursing women?

Food and Drug Interactions

Food can influence the effectiveness of certain medications, so you should ask your doctor if you should take your medication with meals or on an empty stomach. The issue often is whether the drug has any potential to irritate your stomach; if you take your medication with your meals, it will reduce the likelihood of stomach upset. Your doctor also may encourage you to take medication with meals to slow its absorption. Drugs taken on an empty stomach are more rapidly absorbed, which can also be important.

Certain foods may affect the action of the drug you are taking. For example, vitamin K is involved in the body's production of natural blood-clotting substances. If you are taking the anticoagulant Coumadin your doctor may instruct you not to eat large amounts of foods rich in vitamin K (cabbage, cauliflower, spinach, and other leafy green vegetables), or he may have you eat basically the same amount each day (see page 244). Summer splurging on green salads may actually affect your Coumadin need.

Some dietary changes can help make certain medications more effective, even too effective. A few years ago, an elderly woman being treated for congestive heart failure was referred to me and hospitalized with arrythmia, mild diarrhea, a general loss of appetite, and visual disturbances. She was monitored in the intensive-care unit because of her arrhythmia.

I learned that she recently had been diagnosed with congestive heart failure and had begun taking Digitoxin, a digitalis drug, to improve the force of her heartbeat. For several years prior to her diagnosis of congestive heart failure, she also had been taking a diuretic for treatment of hypertension. During this time—and for her own reasons—she severely restricted her intake of salt, although the action of the diuretic made that effort largely unnecessary. What she did not know was that the diuretic was slowly depleting her body of potassium, which was further aggravated by

66

her low-salt diet because potassium loss is directly related to the amount of salt we eat. Potassium is necessary to proper heart function. The increased ratio between her dropping potassium levels and her medication led to digitalis toxicity. Once I replaced her thiazide diuretic with a potassium-sparing diuretic her symptoms ceased and she quickly recovered.

Finding the Right Dose

When first using almost any heart drug, it is important to reach the appropriate blood level of the drug gradually, without risking adverse reactions. Anticipating drug reactions is always prudent, so unless it's an emergency, I start my patients with smaller dosages than the standard recommendations, especially beta blockers and antihypertensives. A potential adverse reaction to certain beta blockers is a constriction of the bronchial tubes. Even Lopressor, which is a B1-selective drug and thus should not affect the lungs, can occasionally cause bronchial constriction and wheezing in some patients. It is imperative for people with a history of asthma to notify their doctor before taking the drug. If the patient has forgotten to tell the doctor about any childhood wheezing, a standard initial dose of the drug might produce some breathing difficulties. Consequently, although the smallest prepared dose of Lopressor is 50 mg, I would prescribe only 25 mg—I have the patient break the tablet in half. Any resulting breathing difficulties will be minor and easily corrected. Another possible adverse reaction to beta blockers is that a full dose can cause some patients' hearts to beat very slowly. Beta blockers—characterized as the "penicillin of cardiology," since they are used for so many purposes—can also cause problems with the libido, sleep, and circulation in the legs. If you or your doctor discovers a problem with an initial low dose of the drug, it can be further reduced, or your doctor can change you to another medication altogether.

Titration

The process by which your doctor slowly increases a drug dosage until the required level is reached is called *titration* (the French word *titre* means "standard"). To titrate is systematically to estimate how much of a specific drug is needed to treat your symptoms successfully and safely.

If your problem is hypertension, the physician will check your blood pressure and, of course, any untoward side effects. If you have angina, the doctor will watch to see what dosage makes your symptoms of angina less frequent, less intense, and shorter in duration. If your problem is arrhythmia, the titration would be influenced by any evidence of palpitations. Your doctor can use a Holter monitor to measure your heartbeat for at least 24 hours as an effective means to help titrate a new antiarrhythmic drug.

Titrating some drugs, digoxin or certain other antiarrhythmic drugs, requires blood testing to safely establish what is an effective level to maintain. Titrating an anticoagulant such as Coumadin would call for testing your blood's clotting ability twice during the first week and once a month after you were titrated and stable.

There are exceptions, of course, to starting gradually on your medications. If you are suffering acutely from a disease, such as dangerously high blood pressure or very bad angina, your doctor will start off with a higher dose than normal. In such an instance, your doctor's concern is that he may be "under treating" what may be an emergency. Any risk of a high dose is offset by the fact that you need prompt treatment. He certainly doesn't want you to have a stroke or heart attack because he was being too cautious about avoiding side effects from the medication.

Pro-time (PT)

Pro-time (PT) is a measure of blood's clotting ability: how long it takes for bleeding to stop. To determine your PT, your doctor draws a sample of blood, mixes it with a clotting agent, and measures the time it takes to coagulate, or thicken. The standard control is approximately 10 seconds, so if your PT time is 15 seconds, your blood is considered 1½ times control. Your doctor may order a pro-time to determine the effective dose of a particular drug, such as Coumadin.

Coumadin and Pro-time

If you are taking the anticoagulant drug Coumadin your doctor will probably measure your PT twice during the first week of use to determine the drug's effectiveness and the right dosage for you. As with many other drugs, the initial dose of Coumadin may vary depending upon need. The standard first dose is 10 mg for the first couple of days, until your PT is brought under control; then a specific amount of the drug is prescribed to maintain an appropriate PT. That stabilizing amount may be as much as 10 mg daily for one person, and as little as ½ mg for another.

The anticoagulant drug Coumadin has been used for a long time for the treatment of blood clots, and it has two different reputations. For years following its introduction in 1954 it was perhaps the most popular "blood thinner" prescribed. When initially introduced, the dosage of Coumadin was frequently high enough to produce easy bruisability and hemophilialike symptoms. Now, however, Coumadin is once again becoming more widely used because doctors have discovered that the symptoms of excessive bleeding are dose-related: in the past many patients who developed adverse symptoms were being overdosed. Doctors were keeping their patients' blood levels at 2 and 2½ times normal pro-time and thus were creating significant bleeding problems. Now, doctors use Coumadin to keep blood levels at about 1½ times normal.

Even so, there's still a risk of bleeding with long-term use of the drug: Statistics indicate a 7 percent incidence of a major bleeding requiring a transfusion, and 2 to 3 percent incidence of a major intestinal or cerebral bleed, if the drug is taken in high doses over the course of a year. I believe that if the drug is used in moderation and with careful monitoring, it can be a reliable and effective anticoagulant.

Still, while taking the drug you have to be sensitive to signs of bleeding, such as bloody gums while tooth brushing, shaving nicks that heal slowly, or unusual bruising. If these symptoms appear, tell your doctor on your next visit. On the other hand, if you have any signs of pathological bleeding, such as coughing up blood, blood when you blow your nose, or blood in your urine or black and tarry stools, do not wait until your next office visit, but notify your doctor immediately.

When your doctor sees you, he should examine your blood to learn its pro-time, the rate at which it is coagulating. Furthermore, depending upon the symptoms, he should also examine you for any secondary cause for the bleeding, such as an underlying lesion or tumor. This evaluation for secondary causes should be done even if your blood is indeed found to be too "thin."

I know of a patient taking Coumadin who complained to his cardiologist that he was coughing up blood and feared that his blood was too "thin." It was determined that his PT was, indeed, much too high, but when his doctor had the patient's lungs x-rayed, he also discovered a very small previously undetected tumor. The bleeding from the lung was actually due to the tumor.

The small capillaries on the surface of a lung tumor will occasionally break and release small amounts of blood. In the early stages of the tumor's growth, the amount of blood released is so small that it usually goes unnoticed. In this case, in the presence of high blood levels of anticoagulant, the tumor bled so much more that it gave away its hiding place. The anticoagulant permitted the small tumor to be located much sooner than it would have been otherwise, and the patient had the growth removed and recovered quickly. The use of Coumadin has also uncovered small tumors or cysts in the kidneys or bladder when patients complained of blood in their urine. A urologist identified these problems and corrected them.

Combination Drugs

Combination drugs are drugs prepared together in fixed dosages and taken as a single pill. The advantages of a combination drug are convenience and cost: purchased in combination the drugs are less expensive than if purchased individually, and it's easier to take only one pill than two. The disadvantage is that they are fixed dosages and cannot be used until the doctor knows what individual dose of each drug is best for you. It is best to adjust the dosage of each drug separately. If, fortuitously, there is a combination pill in the correct formulation for your needs, your doctor will replace your separate pills with the combination pill.

A doctor that uses a combination drug without titrating is jumping the gun. If you began your therapy with a combination drug and developed symptoms related to the medication, you and your doctor might not know which ingredient in the pill was causing the side effects. It's also better to titrate "up" than "down," whether you're being treated for angina, hypertension, or arrhythmia. Your doctor can always back off once you've reached the upper limits of needed medication or when you develop symptoms. Once you develop symptoms from a high dose of a combination or single drug, you frequently have to discontinue it, or at least reduce its dosage to a point that it may become ineffective. Another problem I find is that patients who have had an adverse reaction to a high dose usually don't want to take that medication ever again—at any dose. In some ways, I don't blame them.

Side Effects

By and large, if you follow your doctor's instructions your heart drugs will do what they were intended to do, but no therapeutic drug, whether it's aspirin or a beta blocker, is entirely without potential side effects. There's unpredictability as to how a patient will respond to a particular drug, for we each have our own level of sensitivity. A drug may be safe in one patient and distressing in another. If you have any unacceptable side effects, inform your doctor.

When it comes to new patients' medication histories, I usually find two types of patients: those who don't give much thought at all to possible drug side effects, and those with extreme fear about them. In all cases, I try to assure them that any symptoms people experience while taking these drugs are usually temporary. If they persist or become serious, we can always change the dosage or the drug.

You can exercise some control over possible undesirable drug reactions by asking your doctor or studying the drug profiles in the second part of this book. There you will find detailed information on common side effects—as well as many uncommon and even rare side effects attributed to more than 90 different kinds of heart drugs. Each drug profile describes steps to take to mitigate their effects.

Learning some of the potentially serious reactions, including those that may occur only after a few months of use, can be helpful, even though the vast majority of these reactions are statistically insignificant. Should any of these minor or serious side effects occur, you will be in a better position to judge whether they require immediate action or can be generally ignored, unless they persist. For example, the dry cough that commonly results from taking Capoten is better tolerated when you don't confuse it with symptoms of an impending cold or heart failure.

Physicians' Desk Reference (PDR)

If you wanted even more comprehensive information about side effects, the *Physicians' Desk Reference* (PDR) lists all the side effects experienced during the initial evaluation period mandated by the Federal Drug Administration for all drugs.

Published annually, the PDR is the standard volume doctors consult for basic information on medications. Among other data, the PDR makes recommendations for every prescription drug sold in this country, including the dose with which most patients should begin treatment, at what levels and intervals any increases should be made, and the maximum safe amount to use. The standard recommendations published in the PDR are based on results drawn from a sample population of patients who have used the drug, both sexes and all ages.

The PDR lists only FDA-approved applications and not the expanded uses many drugs have. For example, for many years the FDA recognized Inderal as effective only for hypertension, yet many cardiologists were using it successfully in the treatment of angina years before this use was officially approved.

Your doctor also gathers information about new drugs and their applications from conferences, lectures, seminars, journals, and drug representatives. *The Medical Letter* is a newsletter physicians subscribe to that provides biweekly updates on new drugs and new approaches to treatment.

If you are interested in learning more about the medications you are taking, a copy of the PDR and other similar publications should be found in your local library or bookstore.

Paradoxical Drug Reactions

Heart drugs are not letter-perfect in suppressing all symptoms at all times. In the course of your drug treatment, your symptoms could recur. This could be caused by a change in the status of your disease or a problem with your medication related to drug metabolism and tolerances. Another cause of recurring symptoms could be *paradoxical* side effects, which are symptoms that are drug-related but seem to suggest a worsening of the disease.

Knowing from the outset that your medications could produce contradictory complications can be very helpful. Some antiarrhythmia medications, such as procainamide, mexiletine, and quinidine, can, paradoxically, cause or increase the very symptoms the drug is designed to eliminate. Digoxin, one of the more common cardiac drugs used for congestive heart failure or arrhythmias, has a narrow toxic therapeutic window, meaning that just a small excess can promote arrhythmias.

REPORTING YOUR DRUG'S
EFFECTIVENESS

Visits to your doctor have a two-fold purpose: Your doctor can tell you how you're progressing, and you can tell the doctor how you're progressing. Your cardiologist may want answers to some of these questions:

1. Did you have fewer symptoms?
2. Did you have any side effects to the medication?
3. Did you feel that the effect of the medication didn't last as long as the time interval to the next dose?
4. Was the medication more troubling for you at different times of the day?
5. Did your symptoms change in their severity or duration?
6. Did you have stomach problems? Was it gastritis, nausea, diarrhea, or constipation?
7. Did your episodes of angina decrease in frequency or severity?
8. Do you get light-headed when you stand up, how often, and how soon does your head clear?
9. Has the medicine affected your libido or sleeping habits?
10. Was the dosing schedule difficult to follow?
11. Are you planning on becoming pregnant soon?

I recommend that you keep a diary, at least during the first three to six months of therapy (see "Keeping a Cardiac Diary," page 83). You may not remember all these questions under the pressure of the restricted office visit. I also believe that without a record there is a tendency for some people to report only good news, as if bad news might disappoint the doctor and possibly worry the patient, too. The diary should contain the name of each medication and exact dosages. To avoid (rare) mistakes by your pharmacist, you can carefully check to see you have received the correct drugs and dosages after you have been given the medications and before you leave the pharmacy.

Pro-arrhythmic symptoms are always distressing, but you will be a little less anxious if you know they are produced by your medication and not your disease. I know of patients who despaired that the return of their palpitations meant their condition was deteriorating. One patient compounded her problem by taking two tablets instead of one of the medication she took to stop her palpitations. Instead of reducing the palpitations, the overdose increased them and placed her at still greater risk of a toxic or fatal response. A call to her cardiologist straightened out the confusion.

FOUR
....
Compliance

Noncompliance—not following the doctor's orders—is a major problem in health care today. Studies indicate that as many as one-third of all postcardiac patients fail to fully comply with their recovery program during its first year, and half fail after two years. Many theories have been proposed to explain why so many people fail to comply with their health-care directives. The reasons range from insufficient information about their disease to insufficient motivation. Whatever the reason, if you do not follow the guidelines established by your health-care provider, it ultimately slows your recovery and, in some cases, may bring it to a halt.

The challenge for most cardiac patients is not restricted to taking their drugs as prescribed—although for some even that's a struggle. The area of greatest difficulty is life-style changes. Most of my patients find it difficult significantly to alter their eating habits, eliminate behavior that causes stress, or maintain regular habits of exercise. At the same time, it's my experience that virtually all of my postcardiac patients who were once addicted to cigarettes eventually quit smoking, I suppose because it was easier for them to see smoking as a lethal risk factor only after they had a heart attack. Thus, as elusive as it often is, motivation may be the crucial link to successful compliance.

Even though no doctor can predict in advance which patients will fail to follow instructions, we do know that noncompliance occurs far more often among patients who don't understand the disease or their doctor's directions, or don't feel free to tell the doctor everything related to their care. Admittedly, in some cases the doctor has failed to properly instruct the patient as to the importance of the treatment; in others, the patient did not listen or, for a variety of reasons, grew inattentive over the months or years of treatment.

My recommendation is that you select an annual review period with your cardiologist in which you ask the doctor *any question* you have concerning your past year's treatment. Of course, I don't mean you must defer all questions until this annual review. When you have a question about your health care, you should seek an answer at the time you have the concern. But a scheduled period of review has several distinct advantages for me as a doctor: It makes a statement that all health-care relationships benefit from a review; it encourages patients' confidence in their rights as patients; it demands that they as patients look at all the personal issues that affect their health care; and finally, it's usually an occasion to celebrate successful existing treatment.

The reasons for noncompliance are perplexing—especially among people who have a life-threatening diseases. We'll talk in this chapter about some of the issues that appear to affect compliance and some measures that might help you remain more deeply involved in your treatment.

Understanding Your Illness and Medication

You are statistically a candidate for noncompliance if you do not reasonably or completely understand why you are taking a drug, or if you do not know what potential effect the drug might have on your body. Take, for example, nitrates. These drugs, prescribed for the treatment of irregular heartbeats or arrhythmia, can cause terrible headaches. If, while taking this drug, you suffered headaches for the first two weeks and did not know that Tylenol or one aspirin a day could solve this largely temporary problem, you might become discouraged and stop taking the medication, or at least not take it regularly. Many of my patients have stopped their drugs for lesser reasons.

When patients experience what they believe are unexplained side effects from their medications, they become impatient with their cardiologists and feel a little less confident under their care. I have heard patients actually complain that they thought their doctor was trying to kill them when unexpected side effects made them especially uncomfortable. Strong language, but the sentiment is understandable. When patients are not prepared for the potential side effects of their drugs, they often take it upon themselves to change their medications—and their physicians, too.

The drug Calan (verapamil) was prescribed to a 54-year-old corporate executive who had been a hypertensive patient in the hospital. Within a week, the drug started to irritate his stomach and he reduced his dose by about half. When he returned to his own doctor for his monthly visit he failed to tell him that he had cut his dosage. Because his blood pressure was high, this doctor increased the dosage, not realizing the patient had actually reduced it. Within two weeks, the patient called to say that he thought he was having heart failure because he was dizzy and weak and his heart was "barely beating."

The higher dosage of Calan was slowing his heart rate, an adverse reaction associated with an overdose of the drug. If this patient had confided in his doctor that he had reduced his original dosage, the problem might never have occurred. Once his doctor reduced the elevated dosage, the patient ceased to have any symptoms.

Another patient of mine unexpectedly brought his wife with him to one of our routine office visits. When she asked to sit in on the consultation, I didn't object. The reason for her presence became readily obvious. At one point, when her husband said everything was fine, his wife chimed in: "Don't say that because I know you had pain yesterday. How can you say everything is fine?" He responded by saying it was not important. Then his wife told me that he had taken three nitroglycerin tabs in the last two days. When I asked him if that was true, he said, "I thought it was only one or two, and besides, they were only minor chest pain episodes."

I soon learned that this very sweet but overaccommodating man believed that being a good patient meant he should not bother his doctor with anything but an emergency. He also did not want me to feel I was failing him in his treatment. Finally, he felt it was unmanly to annoy someone with his fears. These are three serious obstacles to effective treatment.

I reemphasized the importance of his treatment and his communicating with me. I also told him that throughout the early stages of his treatment his drug regimen would probably require some adjustments before we would arrive at a correct regimen for him. As this very pleasant couple left, I asked him to call me in a few days and let me know how the new adjusted medication was working—whether the news was good or bad. He seemed relieved that he had more than permission to call—he had an obligation.

Symptomless Diseases and Compliance

Noncompliance often occurs with heart ailments that produce few, if any, symptoms. Most people first become aware of their heart disease when they experience pain or discomfort, most often in the area of the chest, but also in the stomach, back, neck, or jaw. Other patients, though, have no such warning signs and may have no history of symptoms. This can happen with "silent ischemia" or hypertension (see page 81).

It's one thing to be told, after you have had your blood pressure taken or had a stress test, that you have symptoms that suggest heart disease. It's quite another to be taken to the hospital in acute pain because the disease has progressed to a critical state. When patients first learn about their hypertension or silent ischemia they are generally surprised, sometimes disbelieving, whereas patients who experience a painful heart attack are always initially filled with fear and dread. This generally explains how these different sets of patients respond to treatment: the patient with the symptomless disease is far less likely to comply with the prescribed health-care regimen than the patient who has had a traumatic experience. Perhaps it is only human that we are more likely to be inattentive toward treatment if our illness has no physical or distressing symptoms. Yet a counterobservation might be that someone with a serious and largely symptomless ailment would wish to be all the more vigilant because it is hidden and potentially lethal.

Added to the problem of compliance is the fact that the treatment for these symptomless diseases may require lifelong treatment, which may produce side effects. For some people, not to be promised a future cure may be discouraging. It's important to stress that both silent ischemia and hypertension can usually be well managed with little long-term discomfort—if medication is taken as prescribed.

Another compliance issue associated with silent heart disease is that the *treatment* may cause the patient discomfort. Many patients complain of feeling worse *after* they take their medications. After they develop even mild side effects, such as fatigue or depression, they ask, "What am I doing this for? Hypertension didn't bother me until I began treatment for it. My problem is not hypertension but the drugs I'm taking."

This kind of reaction usually can be resolved, or even avoided, if you understand the disease process, the importance of the medications, and their potential for side effects. In most cases the drug reactions are short term, whereas the benefits are long term.

A single warning is not always enough to prevent noncompliance. Although I explain the nature of the disease, what the drugs are designed to accomplish, and the fact that the medications might make the patient feel temporarily dizzy, excessively

SYMPTOMLESS DISEASES: SILENT ISCHEMIA AND HYPERTENSION

"Silent ischemia" is a disease in which the blood flow to the heart is insufficient or obstructed. Usually when your heart is not receiving enough blood and oxygen, it causes pain or angina pectoris. In some instances, however— possibly 25 percent—the heart can be deprived of an adequate amount of blood but provide no clinical symptoms or warning signs. The lack of recognition of the symptoms of cardiac ischemia may be due to altered pain thresholds, symptoms thought to be related to the stomach or musculo-skeletal system, or the fact that less heart muscle is affected. The problem, usually discovered accidentally during a stress test, or from an abnormal electrocardiogram (ECG), is treated much the same as regular angina.

Hypertension can also be symptomless because it may take many years of mild hypertension to develop organ damage; labile hypertension is episodic and may manifest only during physical or emotional stress, but may be normal when measured at rest in the doctor's office.

---

tired, or even a little depressed, only one out of ten patients complains of side effects, usually minor. This rate is similar to that of people taking a harmless placebo. When I ask them to tell me what they think the treatment is trying to accomplish, they often cannot. At that point we sit down and talk again about what they genuinely do not understand about the disease process, why the drug is prescribed, and how it works. I'm convinced that noncompliance would eventually occur if we didn't have this conversation before their first complaint about specific side effects.

Memory and Noncompliance

Even when patients want to cooperate with their treatment, a major problem for busy people is remembering to take their medications when scheduled. The following are some simple suggestions that might make taking your medications easier.

• If you take medications several times a day, say four, ask your pharmacist to divide your pills (if it's a large number) into four small vials. Place the vials at various locations in your home; when you see them, you'll be reminded to take the pill. For example, put your morning dose on the bathroom sink or the breakfast table, your noontime or afternoon dose in your car or office, and your bedtime dose on the night table.

• Some of my patients use an alarm clock, alarm watch, or a small calculator with an alarm to remind them of their medication schedule. It's also best to create a drug regimen around natural breaks in the day, such as your meals, unless it is prescribed *not* to take them with food. If that is the case, take some other predictable points in your day that are easy to remember.

• Elderly people who may be confused about which medicine and what dosage to take can be assisted by having a nurse or relative put all their morning, afternoon, and evening pills in separate, clearly marked small vials or cups.

• From a safety point of view, always check what the doctor has told you to take, and compare it with what the pharmacist has given you. Usually pharmacists are extremely careful; they will give you exactly what your doctor has prescribed. If you have any questions, ask the pharmacist, who may know more about when in relation to meals to take the medication, or drug interaction, than your physician does. Pharmacists frequently have all your drugs on a computer, and they can automatically cross-check for adverse interactions.

• The best drug regimen is once a day rather than three or four times a day, because it's easier to remember to take medications at one specific time rather than several times a day.

Consequently, after a several months of effective use of your medication, ask your doctor if she can prescribe a single long-acting dose to simplify your schedule. Early in the treatment she will titrate to the right dosage, and if you get a side effect, it will be short-lived. Be aware, side effects of long-acting doses will last longer.

Keeping a Cardiac Diary

I always ask patients to keep a cardiac diary. A diary is useful for recording dates, times, dosages, and reactions that might be easily forgotten or not accurately recalled, especially under the pressure patients feel in a doctor's office. Not only can it reveal details that I could not possibly learn on my own, it might also reveal patterns in the occurrence of these symptoms that could prove to be important. A sample patient diary is shown on page 87. (Also see the blank "Cardiac Diary" chart on page 275.)

If my patients complain of chest pains, it's very helpful if I have an accurate record revealing the exact time and duration of the pain over the previous weeks. I would also want to know what precipitated the chest pain, such as heavy exercise or a full meal, and what, if anything, relieved it, such as lying down or bending over. Most cardiologists find a relatively accurate record of such details—even symptoms the patients did not believe were associated with their heart disease—immensely helpful.

On numerous occasions, patient diaries have allowed me to accurately determine that a drug was too weak or too strong or was the wrong drug altogether. One patient told me confidently that he had all his recurring angina pain under control through the use of his medication. But when I examined his diary, I saw that he had been gradually increasing the use of his medication over the preceding two months. He didn't realize it himself until we counted the number of tabs he had taken during an earlier two-month period. When I examined him I discovered evidence that his symptoms were growing more severe and more frequent and that they were lasting longer, necessitating more medication.

In the diary of another patient taking nitroglycerin tabs for angina, I also noted an increased use of medication. In this case, however, it was an unintentional misuse of the drug. The diary showed that this overly anxious patient was taking the drug for symptoms he thought were associated with his coronary pain but were later proved to be unrelated to his disease.

Another example of the value of keeping a diary concerns your diet. If you are being seen for hypercholesterolemia (high cholesterol), and you present a diary record of the food you have eaten for the prior two weeks, the doctor can go through your notes and possibly determine whether the problem is caused in part by your diet. Generally your doctor will recommend medication as a form of therapy only when changes in your diet are unable to lower your dangerously high levels of cholesterol.

In my view, a good diary communicates more than just dates, times, and dosages for the benefit of your doctor. I have seen again and again that sharing a detailed record of treatment and recovery can personalize the relationship between the doctor and patient because it underscores the reality that a *person* is being treated, not a *disease*. Treatment takes place within the daily routine of our lives, whether we are young or old, men or women, letter carriers, housewives or -husbands, salespeople, or executives. The activities of our lives greatly influence the effectiveness of our drugs, our diets, and even our willingness to comply with our treatment. There is an intimate relationship between our psyche and our health. Recognition of stress events that can be avoided or dealt with can sometimes improve our general health and even reduce our medication requirements. A good diary can help make that point evident to both doctor and patient.

Some patients feel comforted or in greater control of their health care if they are able to offer day-to-day details of their treatment for their doctor's close evaluation. I also believe that many patients are simply surprised by how they see their own habits of health care differently when reading a record of them to their doctor weeks or months later.

A few years ago I was treating a woman in her midforties, an advertising executive, for mitral valve prolapse (MVP). Despite her medications, she said she still had occasional panic attacks. Her diary told a fuller story.

Each day she drove by herself to work. By the time she reached her exit, her heart had begun to race so that she routinely would pull over to the side of the road. Before she reached the office, she might stop two or three times to rest. On top of that, once or twice during the day she would go to the women's lounge and lie down. Interestingly, her diary demonstrated that she suffered no such symptoms on the way home, in the evening, or on the weekends. Only after I pointed this pattern out to her did she realize that her anxiety about her work posed a genuine threat to her health. Only when presented with her own one-month record did she finally understand what had to be done: find a less stressful job. As she herself said, "My diary doesn't lie."

Her denial made it hard for her to come to grips with her situation. In fact, she told me that first reading the diary made her feel shame, especially over how little control she had over her situation. I believe that the diary actually permitted her to tell me something she could not, that she was afraid and desperate, and that if it were not for the diary, she might have continued in denial until she became seriously ill.

This woman became a splendid patient once she understood— thanks to her diary—that her recovery required more than a faithful reliance on her medications. She eventually accepted the necessity of making specific life-style changes, including changing jobs.

Another patient, also in his forties, kept the most complete diary of any patient I've ever treated. This man, who had had a heart attack 15 months before, taught accounting in a local community college and was a compulsive record keeper. When he began his diary, he scrupulously recorded his blood pressure three times a day. This meant that between visits he recorded his blood pressure 100 to 200 times. I always looked at each page, and his pressure always varied a little but within an acceptable range for him. The major dividend of his diary was the confidence he gained from it as a patient. Before I had him keep a diary, he would call me once or twice a week about a "worrisome" 5-millimeter change in his blood pressure, even though I told him that occasional changes in blood pressure readings were to be expected and were not the same as persistent high blood pressure. Once he started keeping a daily record, however, everything changed.

The ritual became that at each visit I would read "the record" and then pronounced that everything was fine. With repeated visits, this little exercise confirmed his confidence and competence at making a self-assessment and assured him that his health care was being effectively managed. It wasn't so much that he didn't understand the difference between situational changes in blood pressure versus hypertension as that he wanted me *to see* the pattern of changes. Only then could he accept my reassurance.

In this age of the FAX machine, there may be no need to present your doctor with a three-month record, which your doctor may not have time to study during your office visit. If you feel the need to furnish copious notes every two weeks or to send data at any time you believe something is wrong, you might make arrangements to FAX your notes. If nothing requires immediate attention, the doctor need not respond and you can wait in confidence for your next scheduled visit.

In summary, I'm always encouraged when patients pull out a written record or diary after I've asked them a question about their disease or use of medication. Rightly or wrongly, I immediately assume these patients are taking the enterprise of their health care more seriously than those who keep no record. Not that patients without a diary are necessarily less thoughtful or earnest about their health care; but I've been helped too often by what I've found in a patient's diary not to have a preference for patient record keeping.

SAMPLE PATIENT DIARY

Date: 4/3/91

Time: 5:30 p.m.

Symptom: Discomfort in lower chest near breast bone.

Trigger: Brought on by hectic telephone call from a client.

Relieved by (other than medication): Tried to lie down, but it didn't work. So I took my nitroglycerin medication.

Medication (time and dosage): 2 NITRO-DURO TABS (5:45 p.m.)

Duration (when symptom ceased): Ceased 4 minutes after taking 2 NITRO-DURO TABS. Total duration: 20 minutes from when it came on to when it stopped.

Associated symptoms: Pulse rate was high (I didn't measure it) and, for a few moments, I thought I was going to faint.

Doctor comments: This is the third time he has taken NITRO TABS in two weeks, more often than he had in the past two months, according to his diary. The good news was that each time he took the drug, it was effective immediately. Hence, I wanted to learn if he thought he was starting to use his medications prematurely. In the past he had worried about the side effects of his medication and had delayed too long before taking Nitros.

The near-fainting episode was also something that needed to be considered, as it could mean that his disease was getting worse, or could be a side effect of taking 2 Nitros in rapid succession. Advised him to take a 3- to 5-minute interval between nitros, otherwise hypotension (dizziness or fainting) might develop.

Since it was his first reported fainting spell, and he had been under great stress in his business during this period, I told him to call me and come in if he had another one. He need not wait for an appointment. I told him to stop drinking coffee and start taking 10-minute stress breaks in the morning and afternoon.

The next week he came in saying he had dizzy spells, so I examined him carefully and placed him on a Holter monitor. The results were negative: There was no change in his condition and no correlation between his dizzy spells at peak stress periods at work and any cardiac arrhythmia. He and I have continued to work on reducing the stress in his personal and business life and his episodes have disappeared.

....

FIVE

Diagnostic Tests and Procedures

Over the years, we have learned a great deal about what causes heart disease. The famous Framingham Heart Study, in which the health history of an entire Massachusetts town was monitored by regular examinations and recorded, revealed that a causal relationship exists between our genes, the way we live, and the likelihood of our contracting heart disease. The more risk factors we are exposed to, the more likely we are to have a heart attack.

Who Gets Heart Disease

Risk factors are conditions or behaviors that increase your risk of having a disease. Today most people understand that being overweight, having high blood pressure, and smoking are risk factors creating a greater likelihood of heart attack. Despite improvements in heart disease prevention such as reducing the fat content of our diets, quitting smoking, and taking regular physical exercise, millions of people are still exposed to unnecessary risk factors.

We have also learned that risk factors, in combination, have a multiplier effect. Smokers run a three to five times greater risk of developing heart disease than nonsmokers; overweight people are at a similar increased risk of a heart attack. If you both smoke and have one other risk factor, such as being overweight or having a high cholesterol level, you are considered to be at approximately 16 times greater risk of having a heart attack than with no risk factors at all.

Generally, the major risk factors can be divided into two categories: avoidable, or voluntary, and unavoidable, or involuntary. Voluntary risk factors are usually related to life-style or environment. Involuntary risk factors are age, sex, race, and heredity.

Voluntary, or Controllable, Risk Factors

The most serious voluntary risk factors are cigarette smoking, elevated blood fat levels, obesity, high blood pressure, and a sedentary life-style or lack of meaningful exercise.

Smoking

There is nothing about smoking that is good, even if you smoke only cigars or a pipe. Nicotine, an active ingredient of tobacco, is classified as one of the most toxic of all poisons, and, when inhaled in smoking, it's addicting.

Of all tobacco habits, cigarette smoking is the most ruinous, ranking as our most significant preventable cause of premature death and disability. Cigarette smoking is primarily associated with lung disease, cancer, and cancers of the mouth, larynx, pharynx, and urinary bladder. But smoking is also a major contributor to coronary heart disease.

The nicotine in cigarette smoke causes the adrenal glands to release powerful stimulants that raise blood pressure and cause the heart to work harder. As a result, the heart requires greater amounts of oxygen. In addition, the carbon monoxide of cigarette smoke enters the bloodstream and further decreases the amount of oxygen available in the blood.

Perhaps a more serious consequence of smoking is the increase in the severity of atherosclerosis, which is the buildup of fat deposits on the inner walls of our arteries. The carbon monoxide in the smoke injures the vessel wall in such a way that cholesterol sticks to it more easily, narrowing the passageway of the vessel. If the arteries become narrow or twisted by plaque formation, the blood flow to various organs can be interrupted, causing cell tissue to die. For example, if blood flow to the heart muscle is blocked, angina or a heart attack will occur; if the vessel becomes distorted and slows the blood flow, the blood that is blocked can form a clot, which may lead to a stroke. Smoking may also be associated with an aneurysm, a permanent and abnormal widening or "ballooning," of the aorta or other blood vessels. Once the artery's walls grow weak and begin to stretch, there is the risk that it could eventually rupture, which would be fatal.

Once you stop smoking your risk decreases to some degree almost immediately, and after more than 10 years, your risk of dying from coronary heart disease is statistically about the same as that of a lifetime nonsmoker. Although quitting smoking can be a very difficult effort, each year 3 million people succeed. It's my experience as a cardiologist that proper support combined with proper motivation is the best prescription for success. Of course, everyone has his or her own unique response to smoking: people smoke for different reasons and in different patterns and, most important, have different levels of addiction.

An effective motivation for quitting smoking is the invocation of guilt that passive smoking is dangerous for your household. Additionally, by persisting in the suicidal addiction of smoking you will almost certainly reduce your quality of life and shorten your years. Although this may not be important to you, it's selfish not to consider those who love you and depend on you.

For the first few days after you quit, you may feel irritable, as your body craves the nicotine. Within three days most of the nicotine will have left your body. But withdrawal symptoms will persist for several weeks, since traces of it may remain; beyond that, psychological cravings will continue periodically for months, since smoking has become part of your daily routine in many different ways.

HELPFUL HINTS TO STOP SMOKING

1. Place pictures of loved ones on the outside of your wallet to remind you of them each time you buy cigarettes. Also, slip a photograph of a loved family member inside the cellophane wrapper of the cigarette pack itself.
2. Do not borrow cigarettes; buy your own.
3. Chew gum or fresh vegetables when craving starts.
4. Open a new pack and mark each cigarette from 1–20. Then mix them up and put them back in the pack. You must smoke them in proper numerical sequence. The frustration of finding the next cigarette may reduce your urge. Numbering also assists in your cutting down gradually.

Relapses are more likely to occur during the first few months, and it's advisable to develop various strategies to anticipate when your urge to smoke may surface. Before you quit smoking, think about the occasions and places when you normally have a cigarette. It may not be possible to avoid all those circumstances, but if you can change some features of those situations, it may be easier to resist the urge.

For example, if you are a morning smoker, have some chewing gum (see "Nicotine Gum," page 92) or a glass of water available on your night table and change other features of your morning routine, such as where you drink your coffee. During the day, leave the table as soon as you finish your meal, and have low-fat snack foods available where a smoking impulse may occur, such as at your desk, near the telephone, or in the car. You might also want to temporarily avoid some of the activities that encourage smoking, such as drinking alcohol before meals. Another thought is that when an urge to smoke begins, start an activity that requires the use of your hands, such as washing the dishes, the floor, or the car. Almost any physical exercise, such as getting on the floor and stretching or a yoga exercise, will help you get through the urge.

If past efforts have not succeeded, before you start again consider why you failed. Remind yourself of what you have already learned about how you need to quit. Most ex-smokers did not succeed on their first try, so just remember your commitment to become an ex-smoker. Nothing can replace the need for an abiding commitment to quit smoking and an intelligent program of support, but there are devices and aids that can help.

Low-nicotine cigarettes. The idea that smoking low-nicotine cigarettes is helpful in reducing the harmful effects of cigarette smoke may be illusionary. One reputable study indicated that participants who smoked low-nicotine cigarettes took more puffs, inhaled more deeply, and tended to hold the smoke in their lungs longer. In effect, the hazards these smokers were exposed to were equal to or worse than those for people who smoked high-tar and high-nicotine cigarettes. Coupled with the fact that these smokers also increased the number of cigarettes they smoked, the conclusion of the study was that smoke exposure and carbon monoxide levels increased with smoking low-nicotine cigarettes.

Statistics for lung cancer are even more revealing: Although the tar and nicotine contents of cigarettes fell by half between 1955 and 1975, the incidence of lung cancer among U.S. males increased by 70 percent. Of course, those mortalities may have been influenced by smoking habits prior to the introduction of low nicotine cigarettes, or by other factors, such as poor air quality, but the evidence strongly points to little or no benefits from smoking low-nicotine cigarettes.

Nicotine gum. Nicorettes are a prescription chewing gum that contains a nicotine resin, which is gradually released as the gum is chewed. This gum has been found to be helpful for many smokers when they were trying to quit. To be effective, it should be used under supervision and as part of a larger treatment program.

It may take you a few days to grow accustomed to the spicy taste of the gum, and it may give you slight but temporary indigestion. But the gum can be effective, especially for those whose addiction to nicotine has caused the kind of withdrawal symptoms that made it impossible to quit smoking in the past. In one study, about half of those using the nicotine gum quit smoking, whereas fewer than 25 percent of those chewing a gum without the resin had quit.

Nicotine Patches (Habitrol). Patches, which contain varying dosages of nicotine that is slowly released into the bloodstream, may be effective in weaning people from nicotine addiction. Side effects include allergic skin reactions, exacerbation of heart disease symptoms, delayed healing of ulcers, and interactions with other medications.

Exercise

A sedentary life-style is viewed as a potential risk factor because people who seldom exercise have a somewhat higher heart attack rate. These same people are also more likely to be obese and have higher cholesterol levels.

Many postcardiac patients ask, "Why exercise? It's too late to prevent heart disease with regular exercise now." Regular exercise can't reverse the effects of heart disease, but it can improve the chances for recovery and for a longer and more healthy life. Generally speaking, regular exercise can strengthen your heart so it can pump blood with less effort, which is always important. It also lowers blood pressure, decreases blood fat levels (including cholesterol), may help reduce body weight and body fat, and may even improve the effectiveness of some of your medications. In some cases, it may reduce stress levels and lower blood-sugar levels.

Many of my patients, especially those who seldom exercised before they developed heart disease, have found that regular moderate exercise permitted them to concentrate better, improved their stamina so they did not tire as easily, gave them a feeling of well-being, and renewed their confidence in what their body can do.

To me, "regular exercise" means aerobic exercise for 20 minutes at least three times a week. This type of sustained exercise increases your body's need for oxygen, which strengthens the fibers of your heart muscle and the efficiency of your lungs, and improves the ability of your blood vessels to carry oxygen. Improving the beating strength of the heart muscle means your heart can deliver more blood with each beat or move the same amount of blood with fewer beats. Moderate physical conditioning can lower your heart rate by five beats a minute (unless you're already in great condition), which means your heart would beat approximately 2.6 million fewer times a year.

If you are over 40 and have had any history of heart disease risk factors you should see your doctor about an exercise tolerance, or stress, test (see page 105) before starting an exercise program. Furthermore, no matter what aerobic exercise you choose, start it slowly, especially if it's one at which you had been proficient in years past. Your past proficiency may lead you to try too much too fast. Do not press yourself. Set moderate goals and gradually work up to them. One of the more characteristic precipitants of a heart attack in men under 60 is an uncustomary but intensive period of exercise, when they think they can pick up right where they left off 20 years ago.

If your exercise involves competition, be extra careful about overdoing it. When you play to win, you may not pay attention to your exercise limits and may overexert yourself. A great concern of one patient was that he might not be able to play competitive squash after having a major heart attack and bypass surgery. Slowly, on a regular exercise regimen, he worked himself back to playing squash twice weekly, but now he only plays doubles. And he doesn't overexert himself on every point; if necessary, he leaves the difficult shot to his playing partner.

So don't be in a hurry to get into shape. Any program of regular exercise that cannot be comfortably fit into your weekly schedule is one that you are not likely to stay with; worse, it may encourage you to go at it too intensely on those few occasions when you find time. In addition to tennis, jogging, or swimming, some other suitable aerobic exercises are walking, fast walking, bicycling, and aerobic dancing. During the winter, walking swiftly in a mall or your local park will provide a good workout. Weightlifting should be done only with light weights for toning and not heavy weights for adding bulk muscle. Lifting deadweight may actually strain the heart rather than benefit it. Lifting 20 pounds six consecutive times has more training benefit for your heart than straining to press a 120-pound weight once.

Before you formally begin your period of aerobic exercise, I recommend that you take about five minutes to slowly warm up your muscles, especially by stretching your legs. This is also a good time to quiet yourself if you're upset, because exercising when you are deeply distressed or troubled about something is unwise for heart patients. Also, do not exercise after drinking alcohol or eating a heavy meal, and if you have angina, severe fatigue, dizziness, or any shortness of breath, stop your exercise. First rest; then, if necessary, take your medication.

Following your exercise period, take a similar amount of time to cool down. For example, if you were running, walk slowly for a few minutes until your heart rate and respiration return to relatively normal levels and, then, rhythmically stretch your muscles to reduce the likelihood of soreness. Many patients look forward to their 20 to 30 minutes of private exercise as time to unwind, release anxiety and tension, and perhaps listen to music on a Walkman.

Diet and Cholesterol

Over the years we have discovered that there is a direct link between diet and heart disease. A high-fat diet that produces elevated blood fat levels can influence the likelihood of angina, heart attack, stroke, high blood pressure, and arteriosclerosis.

Cholesterol, a particular type of fat, or lipid, is a waxy substance necessary for a variety of necessary functions in the body, including the building and functioning of all body tissue and maintenance of a healthy nervous system. Almost all of our necessary cholesterol is manufactured in our liver and only a relatively small amount is necessary from our diet. At elevated levels, however, circulating cholesterol can cause a buildup of fatty deposits on the walls of our blood vessels and, eventually, clog them.

When we discuss cholesterol, we must distinguish between several different fats, or lipids: low-density lipoproteins, high-density lipoproteins, and triglycerides. Lipoprotein is a substance formed by combining a protein with the cholesterol; in this form the fat circulates in our blood. Lipoproteins vary in size, weight, and density. Low-density lipoproteins (LDL) pose a risk of coronary artery disease because they tend to form deposits on the walls of our arteries. High-density lipoprotein (HDL), on the other hand, is beneficial in that it acts to remove LDL from the vessel wall and thereby reduces the risk of coronary artery disease. Triglycerides are also blood fats whose high blood levels are associated with problems such as diabetes and atherosclerosis.

SOME DIET HINTS

1. Begin by eliminating certain very rich foods and fried foods.
2. Gradually reduce the number of eggs each week. Substitute "artificial" eggs or use only egg whites.
3. Eat smaller portions: a smaller piece of pie, half of a sandwich, only one slice of bread. Learn how to eat less "bad" foods gradually.
4. Fill up on raw vegetables.
5. Chew sugarless gum.
6. Have a piece of cake one night a week only.
7. When eating in restaurants, ask for broiled fish or low-cholesterol selections.

Radical diets, such as liquid protein or milkshake substitutes, are frequently effective in the short term, but most people begin to regain the weight lost once they eat regularly again. The major reason for the relapse is that the person hasn't learned to modify eating habits and choose the right foods in the correct portion size.

Overeating can have neurotic causes and can be compulsive, involving a drive for immediate gratification or immature psychological dependency. (If you think you have an eating disorder, seek therapeutic help to change your eating patterns. Support groups such as Overeaters Anonymous or Weight Watchers can be effective.)

Don't be frustrated if you occasionally cheat or if the pounds do not "melt" off. As losing weight is a balance of calories taken in versus calories burned off, combining an exercise regimen with your dieting can be beneficial.

Some people inherit a tendency toward abnormal blood fat values, called *hypercholesterolemia* (high levels of blood cholesterol), and some people may also have a genetic disposition to high triglyceride levels. But our diet is the primary cause of elevated blood fat levels and this is where we can often control our cholesterol levels.

If your blood cholesterol levels place you at moderate to high risk of coronary artery disease, your first step is to reduce or eliminate foods high in cholesterol or saturated fats, such as eggs, butter, saturated oils (palm kernel, coconut, and other tropical oils), organ meats, ice cream, and creamy cheeses. (You can get a full list of foods that are high in cholesterol and saturated fats and foods relatively low in fat and/or cholesterol from your doctor, a registered dietitian, or your local chapter of the American Heart Association.) If, after about two months, the diet is unable to bring your cholesterol levels down to a desired level, I would add medication to the treatment, but the diet would not be abandoned.

Cholesterol Screening. Research has shown that the likelihood of developing coronary artery disease increases steadily as blood cholesterol levels exceed 180 milligrams per deciliter, one-tenth liter, of blood. It is advisable to have your total (LDL plus HDL levels) blood cholesterol measured. You should eat nothing and drink only water for 12 hours before your blood is taken.

Desirable total cholesterol is designated as less than 200 milligrams per deciliter, or mg/dl; readings of 200–239 mg/dl are considered *borderline-high*; and 240 mg/dl or more is a *high* cholesterol reading. If your total blood cholesterol level is desirable, you need to have it checked only every four to five years. If your total blood cholesterol level is *borderline-high* and you have two or more heart disease risk factors, or if it is high, you should have a second cholesterol screening performed within a few days or weeks, and then an annual cholesterol screening. The purpose of the second screening is to determine your LDL and HDL cholesterol levels.

Knowing your LDL and HDL levels helps your doctor assess

your risk more completely and plan a treatment program. The higher your LDL cholesterol level the greater your likelihood of developing coronary artery disease. It is the LDL cholesterol, not the HDL, that forms fat deposits that lead to atherosclerosis.

Desirable LDL cholesterol level is designated as less than 130 mg/dl; readings of 130 to 159 mg/dl is considered borderline-high; and 160 mg/dl or more is high. If your LDL cholesterol level is desirable, you need to have it checked only every four to five years. If it is borderline-high and you have two or more heart disease risk factors or if your LDL cholesterol level is high, your doctor will recommend dietary measures to bring the LDL level down. If these efforts fail to bring your level down to acceptable levels, drug therapy may be advised.

Hypertension and dietary salt. Common table salt, or sodium, found in the mineral compound sodium chloride, is a necessary part of our diet. Animals, plants, and humans cannot live without it. But too much sodium can make us ill, and in susceptible individuals, it may be a factor in promoting hypertension.

If your kidneys cannot excrete any unused salt you consume, it is retained in the body. Salt is stored in water, and excess salt leads to additional water being retained in the body to hold the sodium. This adds to blood pressure by increasing the volume of blood circulating.

It can be difficult to reduce the salt in our diet because many of us have developed a heightened taste for it. Furthermore, although we are conscious of the salt we use in cooking and put on our food at the table, much of the sodium in our diet is hidden. Fast foods make a significant contribution to our total daily sodium intake, especially hamburgers, as do processed canned foods (including vegetables), as they tend to be very high in sodium. Manufacturers add sodium compounds in various forms to do a variety of tasks, such as preserve, bleach, enhance flavor, soften or smooth texture, or retard the growth of potential mold in foods. Even over-the-counter medicines such as antacids may contain significant amounts of sodium. So it pays to read labels.

If you have heart disease and your salt consumption should be reduced, your doctor may place you on a low-salt diet. If that's not sufficient to reduce your water retention or high levels of blood pressure, your doctor may also give you a diuretic.

For people who need to have the taste of salt in their food, "salt substitutes" that taste like salt are available. These compounds are usually composed of potassium chloride or some other potassium compound.

In conclusion, if we lead reasonable and moderate lives, exercise sensibly, eat a diet that is relatively low in fat, manage our stress intelligently, have our blood pressure and blood cholesterol checked annually (if we are at risk), and follow our doctor's directives about the proper use of our medications, we are exercising intelligent control over voluntary risk factors in heart disease.

Uncontrollable Risk Factors

Conditions that are beyond our control, such as heredity, age, sex, and race, can place us at an increased risk of heart disease. Although these risk factors cannot be avoided, their more serious effects can be diminished by reducing the overall number of our total risk factors, including controllable ones.

Heredity

Genetic characteristics can strongly influence the nature and timing of a heart attack. A history of premature heart attacks in males in your family under the age of 55—including father, uncle, brother, or first cousins—would point to genetic cause. Most cardiologists can tell you of families they have treated in which several members of different generations suffered from or died of the same type of heart disease, such as severe coronary disease, a congenital defect in the heart, or hypercholesterolemia. Inherited factors can be said to be statistically predictive in identifying people who are susceptible to certain types of heart disease.

Some families share not only genes but also behaviors that could contribute to heart disease. For example, obesity runs in families; and although smoking and alcoholism are not necessarily inherited characteristics, they also appear more often and in more extreme form in some families than others.

Even with inherited and therefore unavoidable risk factors, preventive measures taken early can still reduce the likelihood of their occurrence and, if they do occur, of their harmfulness. You cannot change the cards you have been dealt, but you can change the way you play them. If you know your mother, father, brother, or sister has had a heart attack, or some form of heart disease detected under the age of 55—and this includes diabetes—it's even more necessary that you act to reduce or avoid all risk factors, such as obesity or high blood pressure, that you can control.

Gender

Epidemiological studies indicate that under age 60, men experience a higher incidence of heart disease and higher death rates from heart attacks than women. Beyond the age of 60, however, sex does not appear to be a risk factor. Two explanations for this difference are that men exhibit a higher level of specific risk factors and that women appear to receive added protection from heart disease until they reach menopause possibly from specific hormones. Women who reach menopause very early or have a hysterectomy appear to experience higher incidence of heart attacks. Also, some studies show that women who take birth control pills may increase their risk of heart disease.

A disturbing issue regarding women and heart disease is the claim that women may not be receiving the same treatment for heart disease as men. Two recent studies revealed that women with heart disease were less likely to undergo a *cardiac catheterization* (see page 107) than men. The same studies also found that women were less likely to undergo *bypass surgery* or *angioplasty*, although the heart disease of the women in the study tended to be even more advanced than the men. The fact that coronary heart disease has been thought to be primarily a "man's disease" for so many years may have created a regrettable bias among some physicians and internists who treat heart patients. It's conceivable that some physicians underestimate the severity of heart disease in their women patients and, subsequently, undertreat them.

In response to these studies, and the fact that some doctors were probably trained to take men's heart disease more seriously than women's, the medical community has begun to urge all doctors to reconsider their approach to treating women with heart disease.

In light of this potential bias, I would advise all women patients to be particularly insistent about what they believe is appropriate care for themselves. If you have any symptoms that suggest heart disease, especially chest pains, consult a board-certified cardiologist. In addition to a thorough physical examination you should expect to undergo all appropriate diagnostic testing that a man with similar symptoms would receive. Ask what tests are being considered? If your doctor believes additional diagnostic procedures are not necessary—and they might not be—ask him or her why not. If you are not satisfied with the answer, speak to your doctor about your concern.

Race
It's not clear whether racial differences account for a disparity in the incidence of heart disease among white and black men and the incident of hypertension among them. Statistically, hypertension and other forms of heart disease are several times more common among black men than among white. Furthermore, black men are more likely to die from a stroke than white men of the same age. The reasons are probably complex, and further influenced by cultural factors as well, such as diet and environment. Asians generally have fewer heart attacks than whites, possibly because of diet.

The Elderly and Pregnant Women
The only groups for which heart drugs pose a special risk are the elderly and pregnant women. The problem for the elderly is

related to their slowed metabolism (see page 56) and the danger for the pregnant women is primarily to her fetus.

The elderly. Because we metabolize our food and drugs more slowly as we age, drugs may remain longer in the body, which means their effects last longer. In addition, because kidney and liver function may become impaired with age, the elderly do not always effectively excrete their drugs. For both reasons, the elderly are at increased risk of accumulating toxic levels of a drug in their bodies. Most drugs are metabolized in the liver and eliminated through the action of the kidneys. Consequently, anyone suffering from a liver or kidney disease, such as advanced diabetes, that caused these organs not to perform properly might have difficulty eliminating drugs and would run the risk of toxic accumulation. It is always advisable that the dosage and frequency of the medication prescribed be reduced to the lowest therapeutic level.

Pregnant women. The placenta of a pregnant woman contains a selective barrier that permits nutrients and hormones access to the developing fetus while it screens out many substances that might be harmful to it. Many drugs are considered detrimental to the developing fetus, but unfortunately, the placenta cannot protect the fetus from the effects of many, if not most, drugs the mother might take. Hence, if a pregnant woman must take any drugs whatsoever, it should be under the supervision of a physician. There is a pregnancy code at the end of each drug profile in Part Two of this book that indicates the relative risks of using that drug during pregnancy. The risk categories are explained on page 103.

The most exacting and complex period of fetal development occurs during the first three months of pregnancy. During this period, various medications could threaten the delicate growth of the fetus. Consequently, a pregnant woman should avoid taking certain cardiac drugs during her first trimester. It's also important that a woman carefully monitor whether she has become pregnant while taking certain heart drugs. Some drugs remain in the body for a week or more before being completely eliminated. Hence, if you happen to become pregnant while taking cardiac medication, notify your physician immediately. But do not stop taking the medication without first notifying your doctor, unless you have made previous arrangements as to what to do in such a circumstance.

A drug taken by a lactating woman may show up in her milk. Again, consult your physician concerning the use of drugs during your nursing period. All drug use must be seen as a risk/benefit ratio: the potential health risks to the fetus or nursing child weighed against the possible benefits of the drug to the mother's health.

RISK CATEGORIES OF DRUGS USED DURING PREGNANCY

Category A: *Risk to fetus is remote.* Reliable studies of pregnant women are negative for fetal abnormalities.

Category B: *Risk to fetus is relatively low.* Information from animal studies or reliable studies of pregnant women is negative.

Category C: *Possible benefits of the drug to the mother are thought to warrant use despite potential risks to the fetus.* Information from animal studies may be positive for fetal abnormalities, or information from reliable studies of pregnant women is not available. Use during the first trimester of pregnancy should be avoided whenever possible.

Category D: *Only a serious or life-threatening situation warrants the use of this drug.* Studies of pregnant women or experience with the use of the drug have shown a significant risk to the fetus. The drug should be used only if needed for a serious disease and when other safer drugs have proved ineffective or cannot be used.

Category X: *Use of this drug is contraindicated.* Animal studies or human pregnancy studies or experience with the use of drug have proved positive for fetal abnormalities.

Diagnostic Tests and Procedures

Every person over the age of 40 should have an examination for any signs of hypertension, which involves not just having your blood pressure measured, but a thorough physical examination: examination of your heart, lungs, and eyes; and an evaluation of your blood for kidney function, blood sugar, and cholesterol levels.

If you have no symptoms of heart disease and no significant risk factors, such as a family history of heart disease, a similar screening for hypertension every two years suffices, and annual stress testing and other cardiac tests are probably largely unnecessary. If there are changes in the ECG or you develop chest pain or an arrhythmia during an exercise test, your doctor may recommend a more sophisticated exercise test or an angiogram.

Your physician will recommend further diagnostic tests if he hears with the stethoscope any irregularity of your heart or lungs, if you report suspicious symptoms, if blood tests reveal heart-related problems, or if you have significant risk factors.

The following are brief summaries of some of those diagnostic tests.

Electrocardiogram (ECG or EKG)

The working of your heart produces electrical impulses, and a painless test, called an *electrocardiogram*, has been devised that records this electrical activity. By examining the pattern of electrical impulses, your cardiologist learns how your heart responds to increasing levels of work. There are three types of electrocardiogram: a resting ECG, which measures the heart's activity when no demands are made on it; an exercise ECG (stress test), which measures the heart's activity when increased demand is made on it by exercise, etc.; and Holter monitoring, which is continuous monitoring of the heartbeat for at least 24 hours.

Resting ECG. The resting procedure calls for you to lie quietly on an examining table or bed, while 10 electrodes, which read the various electrical impulses generated by your heart, are attached to your legs, arms, and chest. The electrodes send a series of signals to the ECG machine, which transcribes them onto graph paper in the form of little spikes and depressions. The entire process should take less than five minutes. This resting ECG procedure can reveal if there's any evidence of heart disease, particularly arrhythmia, thick heart muscle, or evidence of a prior heart attack. It cannot predict, however, what may happen in the future, such as a heart attack.

Exercise ECG (stress test). A stress test requires that you exercise so your cardiologist can see how your heart responds to an increased need for oxygen. In this manner, your cardiologist can more easily determine the etiology of your chest pain and the general functioning of the heart. The test can be conducted with a treadmill, which looks like a moving belt. Both the speed and incline change, so you walk or run on different grades. A stationary bicycle (bicycle ergometer) may also be used.

As with the resting ECG, electrodes will be attached to monitor the activity of your heart. In addition, your blood pressure will be closely checked during and after the test. The procedure is painless, but the level of exercise might cause you to feel a little tired. If you should feel excessively anxious, dizzy, or short of breath, or have leg cramps or any chest pain, tell your doctor so the test can be stopped. Your cardiologist may also terminate the test if your blood pressure falls (especially your systolic pressure), if your heart does not respond to the increased work, or if you develop palpitations.

I advise you to prepare for the test as follows: Get plenty of rest the night before; do not drink any coffee, tea, or alcohol the day of the test; eat a light meal and do not smoke or take nitroglycerin medication at least two hours before the test; and ask your doctor about taking any other heart medications that may affect the results of the test. Bring sneakers and comfortable clothing.

Relax and rest for one to two hours after the test. Do not take a hot shower during this period. If necessary, you may take a warm bath about two hours later. Again, should you have any questions regarding the purpose of your stress test, ask your doctor before taking the test.

An exercise stress test is a safe, noninvasive, and inexpensive means of evaluating heart disease. It can uncover specific heart abnormalities, especially among those people at high risk of cardiovascular disease, namely, men over 45 and women over 55 who have high cholesterol, high blood pressure, or a family history of heart disease. It's also useful if you are planning an exercise program following a heart attack or heart surgery.

Stress test results are not always reliable, however. They are not necessarily a reliable indicator of whether you will or will not get a heart attack. Some studies show that exercise stress tests fail to accurately diagnose coronary artery disease 35 percent of the time. The lower your risk profile for heart disease is, the less trustworthy the test may be. One study showed that a majority of people who tested positively, but who had no history of heart disease prior to the test and were in the lowest risk category, had not developed angina or a heart attack when their histories were followed for up to six years afterward.

If you ever have positive results from a exercise stress test, consult a cardiologist. The doctor will give you a thorough examination and, if warranted, conduct more reliable tests, probably a thallium stress test (a test that uses a radioactive substance to outline the heart blood supply and identify any danger zones), an echocardiogram (see next section), or a *catheterization* (see page 107), to determine the presence of any potential abnormality.

Holter monitoring. The Holter monitor is a lightweight, portable ECG that is used to monitor all heart activity over a period of time. For this test, you wear a portable tape recorder attached to electrodes on the chest. Depending on how long a period your doctor wants a continuous graphic tracing of your heartbeat, you might wear the Holter monitor for up to several days—and nights. During that time you would be asked to keep a log or diary of your daily activities, especially the time and activity when you had any symptoms or had to take any medication.

The monitor and your written record or diary will help your doctor determine what correlations exist between the ECG and your activities. It's also useful in evaluating arrhythmias or the need for a *pacemaker* (see page 111). If you complain of rare episodes of palpitations, another test made by a *transtelephonic arrhythmia recorder* might be able to pinpoint the source of your complaint. This is a small recorder that can record 60 seconds of a heart rhythm.

Echocardiogram (Ultrasound)

With the use of ultrasound, your cardiologist can get a detailed "picture" of your heart without ever penetrating your body. This procedure, called an echocardiogram, uses high-frequency sound waves to reflect sound off of the heart. This creates an image of the heart that can be used to evaluate the valve chambers and even blood flow velocity in the heart. The image (which can be heard as well as seen in color) reveals the heart working, including the shape and thickness of the chamber walls of the heart, the functioning of the valves, the contraction of the heart muscle, and the condition of the larger arteries and veins that carry blood into and out of the heart. The test is used to diagnose a variety of heart diseases, such as valve disease (prolapse, stenosis, or regurgitation), heart muscle thickening (hypertension), blood clots in the heart, damage from heart attacks, or congenital abnormalities.

For the test you lie on your back on an examining table. A special jelly is applied to various parts of your body, and a hand-held device linked by a cord is placed on your chest to produce a continuous image on a monitor screen. The procedure is completely painless and takes 45 to 60 minutes.

Cardiac Catheterization

Cardiac catheterization is a diagnostic procedure that is more accurate than an electrocardiogram for measuring the extent of coronary artery disease. It's also referred to as a *coronary arteriogram* or *coronary angiogram* (from the Greek *angeion*, meaning "vessel"). The procedure permits your doctor to see, in great detail, the coronary arteries that bring blood to your heart. Not only can catheterization detect the presence of coronary artery disease and give a view of the extent of the damage, it can also determine whether surgery or a balloon angioplasty (see page 110) might correct the problem.

A catheter is a small narrow tube. It is inserted into an artery, usually in the leg or arm, and guided up the artery, through the aorta, and into the heart. Once the catheter is in the heart, a special radiopaque dye is injected into it to make the inside of the heart visible on an X-ray picture. Once X-rays have been made of the pumping action of your heart, the catheter is placed in each of the openings of the coronary arteries and dye is injected into them. Again, your doctor will be able to see how the dye flows into the arteries. If the arteries do not fill completely with the dye, your doctor will be able to see where the arteries are blocked and to what extent.

Before the procedure begins, the area where the catheter is inserted will be shaved and cleaned with an antiseptic solution. The catheter is very small, so it can be passed into the artery and heart without much, if any, discomfort. However, you will have a warm feeling pass through your body for a few moments when the left ventricle is injected with dye. It's also possible that you might feel a little temporary nausea and, if you suffer from arrhythmia, maybe a few extra or slow heartbeats, too. But these feelings will pass quickly. The procedure takes between one and two hours. A catheterization should be performed at a hospital where at least 500 are done annually, and by someone proficient and experienced who does approximately 200 per year. The radiopaque dye is iodine-based; be sure to inform your physician if you are allergic to iodine or shellfish or have had a reaction to a prior X-ray study. Be sure to get plenty of rest the night before you are to have the test, and do not eat or drink anything at least three hours before the procedure.

Corrective Procedures

If your cardiologist discovers evidence of advanced heart disease as a result of a diagnostic test, or if your heart disease has not favorably responded to other therapy, he or she might recommend one of several corrective procedures such as coronary artery bypass surgery, heart valve surgery, or open-heart surgery. These procedures are frequently done to correct a congenital defect of the heart, to treat an aneurysm (a circumscribed bulging of nonfunctioning heart muscle), to remove tumors, to treat diseases of the aorta, or to control arrhythmias that have resisted treatment. The term open-heart surgery refers to operations in which the breast bone is surgically split and the heart is exposed. While the heart is being operated on, the functions of the heart and lungs are temporarily performed by a heart-lung machine, which oxygenates the blood and pumps it through the body. Coronary artery bypass surgery is considered the most common of all open-heart surgeries.

Coronary Artery Bypass Surgery

Unless the situation is deemed an emergency, surgery is elected only after other treatments or strategies such as medications and dietary and life-style changes have failed.

Coronary bypass surgery is performed when there is a significant narrowing of the blood vessels. The preferred surgical treatment is to "bypass" the blockage by taking a section of an artery inside the chest wall (left internal mammary artery, or LIMA) or a vein from the leg or thigh and using it to create an alternative route around the blocked area of the occluded artery. The LIMA is preferable because it stays open for many more years than vein grafts do.

A bypass procedure, from the first incision to completion, may take up to four hours, though the actual sewing of bypass vessels may take only 20 to 40 minutes. Usually you will require a week to 10 days in the hospital for recovery, the first few days in an intensive-care unit. There, your heart functions and other vital signs will be closely watched. During the next few weeks you will gradually resume normal activities.

Heart Valve Surgery

Valvular surgery is performed if a valve doesn't open adequately (stenosis) or if it leaks excessively (regurgitation). The procedure may be a *valve repair*, especially of the mitral valve. When the blood flow through a valve has been restricted, a surgical procedure, called a *valvotomy*, enlarges the opening and restores proper flow. If the valve cannot be repaired or opened by a valvotomy, it may be replaced by a valve made of animal tissue or a mechanical valve made of plastic or metal. Both valve repair and replacement procedures last several hours and are considered highly successful. As with bypass surgery, following heart valve surgery you will spend a few days in the cardiac-care unit where your heart functions and other vital signs will be closely monitored. During the next few weeks, you will gradually resume normal activities.

Coronary Angioplasty

If a narrowed or blocked artery is the cause of angina or heart attack, one of the procedures designed to restore blood flow through the occluded artery is a *coronary angioplasty*, sometimes referred to as percutaneous transluminal coronary angioplasty (PTCA). The technique, also called "the balloon," takes about an hour and is performed while you are awake.

First you are given a local anesthetic, so a catheter or flexible tube can be inserted into an artery in your leg or arm and guided up into the blocked or occluded coronary artery. A small amount of a dye is delivered through the catheter and an X-ray reveals whether the catheter has reached the precise site of the blockage.

A smaller catheter with a balloon tip is then inserted inside the larger catheter. When this tube reaches the blocked area of the artery, the balloon is puffed up for about half a minute to widen the artery and to improve blood flow. The balloon may be inflated and deflated several times to stretch the walls of the artery sufficiently. You may experience chest pressure during inflations. Once the procedure is completed, X-rays will be taken to see if normal blood flow has been restored. For the next few days, you will be closely monitored.

The advantages of coronary angioplasty over bypass surgery are that the procedure is faster and cheaper and you may be in the hospital for only a few days. Unfortunately, not all lesions are amenable or responsive to PTCA. It should also be noted that angioplasty does not cure the underlying disease that causes the blockage, and frequently people need to have the angioplasty performed more than once. Some studies indicate that as many as 30 percent of all patients who have angioplasty eventually require repeat angioplasty or bypass surgery to correct the continued blockage. You may want to obtain a second opinion on the proper choice of therapy by taking the motion picture film of your catheterization to another physician.

Artificial Pacemakers

If your heart doesn't beat properly—particularly if it is very slow or intermittently slow and fast—and you have fainting spells, blackouts, or periods of breathlessness, your cardiologist might recommend that an artificial pacemaker be surgically implanted to help regulate your heart rhythm. Occasionally, an electrophysiological study (EPS) may be recommended in which catheters are inserted into the heart to test its electrical system. A pacemaker weighs little more than an ounce and a half. Powered by a small lithium battery, it sends out electrical impulses that restore a regular heartbeat. In some cases only the ventricle is paced; in others both the atria and ventricle are paced.

Implanting a pacemaker in your body is considered a minor surgical procedure. In most cases, you receive a sedative to relax you, and the site of the incision is numbed to prevent any pain. A 3- to 4-inch incision is made in the upper chest and the pacemaker is placed in a pocket just under the skin. The entire procedure takes about an hour and most people are out of bed the very next day. If your pacemaker is working properly, you should have few if any symptoms. If the device should need an adjustment, your doctor can make changes from outside the body without surgery. Present-day pacemakers are sophisticated computers that can be re-programmed from an external programmer to maximize your heart's performance. And the lithium battery in most permanent pacemakers lasts about 10 years.

The Decision to Have Surgery

Several reliable studies suggest that too many coronary bypass surgeries—operations for patients with significantly blocked heart arteries—are being performed. The statistics are impressive: Coronary bypass surgery is performed 300,000 times a year in this country and accounts for one out of every fifty dollars spent on health care.

Why are there so many heart operations? For one thing, in recent years cardiologists' reluctance to recommend bypass surgery has been lessened because the technology is far better than it has ever been. But the pressure sometimes comes from patients as well. I told two patients with 75 percent blockage in an artery that they had to curtail their active life-styles and take several medications. Both patients said they did not want to reduce any of their activities. Both men were in their fifties, were avid tennis players, and loved to work out. They said they couldn't face life thinking there was something wrong with their heart or that they might become "cripples." Both men stated firmly that they wanted the kind of medical care that would correct the situation and fully restore them to their "former selves." As eager as they were to take the decisive step toward surgery, I urged them to consider other alternatives: medication and angioplasty.

After impatiently taking medications for only several months, they insisted on a change in their treatment: Instead of open-heart surgery, both men elected to have angioplasty. Before choosing angioplasty or bypass surgery, I told them they should understand what their risks were. Angioplasty procedures eventually fail about 30 percent of the time: The procedure has to be repeated to reopen the same artery or another artery when it becomes closed. And there is also a 5 percent incidence of heart attacks as a result of angioplasty, which may require open-heart surgery. The risk of death from open-heart surgery or bypass surgery ranges from one percent to 5 percent.

Two years after their angioplasty one man required a repeat and the other is doing fine. I was also able to convince them that, to take long-term responsibility for their health, they had to make some permanent changes in their life-style, which would improve the long-term effectiveness of the angioplasty.

Another reason bypass surgery may be overused is that people are being sent to surgery without due consideration of other options. For some cardiologists, surgery may appear to be an easier alternative, especially when they are pressured by patients who persistently call to say that they are having angina and that it's not being adequately controlled by their medication. Some patients may not have been given the right combination of medications or may not have taken their medications properly.

Even patients who continue to have anginal pain while taking maximum dosages are not necessarily candidates for open-heart surgery. A patient may be at risk of angina but not at risk of having a major heart attack. For example, a cardiac patient who has had a first heart attack may have blockage in a blood vessel to an area of the heart already replaced with scar tissue. But other blood vessels to the heart work fine; they have no blood vessel blockage that poses an immediate risk of blocking or breaking down.

Another patient may have a blockage but also has collateral, neighboring branches of vessels that deliver enough blood to the heart so the muscle functions very well and the area is not at risk. Their heart may function perfectly well at rest, but they notice mild angina when they exercise. Their blood flow may even be adequate during mild exercise, except that they may develop anginal symptoms with moderate exercise. Patients with collateral vessels may not benefit as much from surgery as those patients with severe blockages without collaterals.

As you can see, open-heart surgery has become a viable option for certain patients with heart disease, but it is a decision that should be made only after a thorough and thoughtful consideration of all the risks and benefits.

Before Surgery

For several days or weeks prior to heart surgery, your cardiologist may have you on a specific regimen, including medications. In addition, it is best to relax, lose weight if possible, do a little exercise (allowed by your doctor), and, if you still smoke, quit. Nourishing your body and resting it before surgery speeds healing. Exercise is intended primarily to relax the body and reduce any stress you may have in anticipation of the surgery.

After Surgery

The course of recovery from open-heart surgery varies according to the type of surgery and the health of the patient. Generally, bypass surgery requires a week to 10 days in the hospital for recovery and some rehabilitation. The recovery period for surgery to repair or replace an enlarged heart valve is about the same as for a bypass, depending on preoperative function of the heart. In all three instances, your first few days will be spent in an intensive care unit, where your cardiologist or surgeon will monitor your heart functions and other vital signs closely to make sure that they are stable and normal. Your breathing tube will be removed within 6 to 12 hours. Once you no longer require intense constant care you will be moved from the intensive-care unit (ICU) to a "step-down unit."

Your routine there may include specific exercises, such as deep breathing and coughing exercises to clear your lungs of any mucus. Coughing is important because mucus usually collects in the lungs during any major surgery and if it remains it can cause serious respiratory infections such as pneumonia. Even though you may feel some pain when coughing, medication can be prescribed to reduce your discomfort. Coughing will not open the chest incision, which is closed with steel sutures.

Rehabilitation

Once you are out of intensive care, your rehabilitation begins in earnest. When you're strong enough, you'll be helped to the side of the bed. As you begin to move around you will notice that your incisions (stitches in your chest and leg for bypass surgery) become less sensitive. The usual progression goes from sitting on the side of the bed, to sitting in a chair, to walking in your room, to walking in the hall. Specific stretching exercises to reduce internal scarring of the chest-wall incision will begin while you are still in the hospital.

After you leave the hospital, you may still be prohibited from strenuous work, since there may have been prior heart muscle damage or there may still be some blockage in smaller blood vessels. If you've had valve surgery, you may have to take a blood thinner, such as Coumadin, for the rest of your life. If the heart has been enlarged, you may have to take another drug to prevent a recurrence of any rhythm disturbance.

Once the surgeon has done his or her job, the responsibility for maintaining your health is yours. It begins immediately after surgery, and should continue for the rest of your life. Recovery may entail significant but sensible life-style changes, including cessation of smoking, dramatic alterations in your diet, more regular exercise, and loss of weight. People who appreciate the importance of their becoming active participants in their health care almost always recover faster and better and are less likely to have a relapse.

PART TWO

Cardiovascular Drug Profiles

SIX

Diuretics

THIAZIDE-TYPE

Brand Name	*Generic Name*
HYDRODIURIL, ESIDRIX, ORETIC, THIURETIC, MICTRIN	hydrochlorothiazide
ZAROXOLYN, DIULO, MICROX	metolazone
LOZOL	indapamide

LOOP DIURETICS

Brand Name	*Generic Name*
LASIX, AGRO-FUROSEMIDE, MYROSEMIDE	furosemide
BUMEX	bumetanide

POTASSIUM-SPARING

Brand Name	*Generic Name*
ALDACTONE	spironolactone
MIDAMOR	amiloride hydrochloride
DYRENIUM	triamterene

COMBINATIONS

Brand Name	*Generic Name*
DYAZIDE	triamterene and hydrochlorothiazide
MAXZIDE	triamterene and hydrochlorothiazide
MODURETIC	amiloride hydrochloride and hydrochlorothiazide

Diuretics are usually the first type of drug used in the treatment of hypertension, either alone or in combination with another hypertensive drug. Diuretics are popular because they offer comparatively fewer adverse reactions than other antihypertensive drugs and are effective in probably half of all cases of hypertension, and their therapeutic effects last longer.

Not all diuretics are the same, though most are related to the same chemical compound, chloro*thiazide*, which was first introduced in 1958. Diuretics differ generally in their relative potency, the length of their effectiveness, or "duration of action," and their potential side effects. At the same time, all diuretics are similar in two important aspects: They increase the amount of salt and water your body excretes—which is why you pass more urine than is normal during the first few days of drug use—and over time they prevent fluid from reaccumulating in your tissue ("edema"), seen principally as a swelling in your hands, legs, and feet. This makes diuretics especially valuable since they can be used in combination with other hypertensive drugs that have fluid retention as a side effect. Diuretics are also used to treat congestive heart failure, of which edema is a symptom.

Potential risks: Although diuretics are considered the safest of the hypertensive drugs in that they produce the fewest side effects, if used over time they can wash out critical amounts of potassium. Potassium loss (*hypokalemia*) can be a serious problem since it can cause severe fatigue, confusion, depression, and a general weakness in your muscles. Perhaps most important, hypokalemia can cause abnormal heart rhythms. The risk of low blood levels of potassium is higher in people taking certain other hypertensive medications along with the diuretic.

The most commonly prescribed type of diuretics are thiazide types. Your doctor may prescribe these diuretics separately or in conjunction with another antihypertensive drugs that may cause fluid retention. If your blood pressure were not responding adequately to the thiazide, or if hypokalemia became a problem while using it, your doctor can prescribe a less powerful type of drug, called a "potassium-sparing" diuretic, which reduces the likelihood of potassium loss.

A third type of diuretic, called a "loop diuretic," is used when other drugs have failed to bring the hypertension under control or to reduce the edema. These potent diuretics are the fastest-acting of the three types and have a shorter duration of action. Loop diuretics act more quickly on the kidneys, causing you to pass large amounts of urine within a few hours of taking the drug, which can be a major nuisance for some people. These drugs are reserved for hypertensive patients with impaired renal or kidney function. For some people, loop diuretics may be more effective than thiazides because they act on a different area of the kidneys. As they are the most powerful of the diuretics, elderly patients are usually treated with smaller doses.

Two other risks associated with the use of diuretics are increased blood levels of uric acid, which can produce gout in certain people, and increased blood sugar levels, which can cause problems for people with diabetes. But by and large, diuretics are the safest and most reliable of all heart drugs and, when used properly, generally do their job without causing any unacceptable side effects or adverse reactions.

THIAZIDE-TYPE DIURETICS

Brand Name	*Generic Name*
HYDRODIURIL, ESIDRIX, ORETIC, THIURETIC, MICTRIN	hydrochlorothiazide (hy-dro-clor-o-THY-a-zide)

How the Drug Works
By causing the kidneys to increase the flow of urine, the body eliminates more salt and water, which reduces the volume of both

blood and fluid in the tissues of the body, and thereby lowers overall blood pressure.

Purpose
Treatment of hypertension or congestive heart failure.

Dosage
• Hypertension
Adults: Initially 25 to 100 mg taken orally daily in single or divided doses, followed by increases, if needed, up to 200 mg daily in divided doses.
• Edema
Adults: 50 mg to 100 mg taken orally once or twice daily.
Children under 6 months: 12.5 mg to 37.5 mg taken orally daily in divided doses, depending upon body weight of the infant.
Children over 6 months: 37.5 mg to 100 mg in two divided doses, depending upon body weight of child.

Side Effects
Uncommon: Diarrhea, dizziness or light-headedness, headache, loss of appetite, decreased sexual ability, sensitivity to sunlight.

Adverse Reactions
Potassium loss, leading to dry mouth, increased thirst, irregular heart beat, mood changes, muscle cramps, nausea, fatigue and unusual weakness, and a weak pulse. *Rare:* sore throat, fever, stomach cramps, vomiting, blurred vision, unusual bleeding or bruising, yellowing of the eyes or skin.

Drug Interaction
Increases the effects of other hypertensive drugs.
With lithium, it increases risk of toxicity.
With steroids, it increases risk of hypokalemia (low levels of potassium).

Overdosage

If any of the following symptoms develop, a physician should be notified immediately: extreme lethargy, dizziness, confusion, coma.

Comments

Hydrochlorothiazide diuretics belongs to a class of drugs called thiazide diuretics. These drugs, first introduced in the late 1950's, are often used as the first drug in treating hypertension because they are long acting (one dose should last all day) and they produce few side effects. Thiazide diuretics are preferred by many doctors over other diuretics, specifically "loop" diuretics, because they act more gradually on the kidneys and over a longer period of time. This means you may not have to run to the bathroom as frequently while taking thiazide diuretics.

Notify your doctor if you have been taking a monoamine oxidase (MAO) inhibitor drug in the past 14 days, or if you suffer from diabetes; gout; kidney, liver, or pancreatic disease; or an autoimmune disease such as lupus. Your blood and urine will probably be monitored periodically, especially if you have a history of gout, to determine if the drug is effective.

As the drug eliminates salt and water from your body, it may also reduce your level of potassium. Some of the more common symptoms of potassium loss are excessive thirst, dry mouth, unusual weakness, lethargy, stomach cramps, restlessness and irritability. To reduce the likelihood of low levels of potassium, it is recommended that you include potassium-rich foods in your diet, such as tomatoes, bananas, and citrus fruit.

Although you may experience mild diarrhea or an upset stomach, loss of appetite, dizziness, or a sensitivity to sunlight (sunburn), these symptoms should cease as soon as your body adjusts to the medication. If you are taking only one dose each day, it is recommended that it be taken in the morning, preferably after breakfast. If you taking more than one dose, take the last one approximately four to six hours before your bedtime. If you miss a dose, take it as soon as possible. However, if the next scheduled dose is within four hours, do not take the missed dose. At no time should you double up a dose.

Pregnancy

Category D (see page 103). Since the drug appears in breast milk, consult your doctor before you begin breast-feeding.

Brand Name	*Generic Name*
ZAROXOLYN, DIULO,	metolazone
MICROX	(me-TO-la-zone)

How the Drug Works

By causing the kidneys to increase the flow of urine, the body eliminates more salt and water, which reduces the volume of both blood and fluid in the tissues of the body, and thereby lowers overall blood pressure.

Purpose

Treatment of mild hypertension or congestive heart failure.

Dosage

• Treatment of edema
  Adults: 5 mg to 10 mg taken orally once daily.
• Treatment of hypertension
  Adults: 2.5 mg to 5 mg taken orally once daily, followed by increases, if needed, to 20 mg.

Side Effects

Uncommon: Diarrhea, dizziness or light-headedness, headache, loss of appetite, decreased sexual ability, sensitivity to sunlight.

Adverse Reactions

Potassium loss (dry mouth, increased thirst, irregular heartbeat, mood changes, muscle cramps, nausea, fatigue and unusual weakness, and a weak pulse).

Rare: Sore throat, fever, stomach cramps, vomiting, blurred vision, unusual bleeding or bruising, yellowing of the eyes or skin.

Drug Interaction

Increases the effects of other antihypertensive drugs.

With steroids, it increases risk of hypokalemia (low levels of potassium).

Overdosage

If any of the following symptoms develop, a physician should be notified immediately: Extreme lethargy, dizziness, confusion, coma.

Comments

Metolazone, first introduced in 1973, belongs to a class of diuretics called thiazide diuretics. These drugs are often used as the first drug in treating hypertension because they are long acting (one dose should last all day) and they produce few side effects. Thiazide diuretics are preferred by many doctors over other diuretics, specifically "loop" diuretics, because they act more gradually on the kidneys and over a longer period of time. This means you may not have to run to the bathroom as frequently while taking them.

Notify your doctor if you have been taking a monoamine oxidase (MAO) inhibitor drug in the past 14 days; if you suffer from diabetes; or gout; kidney, liver, or pancreatic disease; or an autoimmune disease such as lupus. Your blood and urine will probably be monitored periodically, especially if you have a history of gout, to determine if the drug is effective.

As the drug eliminates salt and water from your body, it may also reduce your level of potassium. Some of the more common symptoms of potassium loss are excessive thirst, dry mouth, unusual weakness, lethargy, stomach cramps, restlessness and irritability. To reduce the likelihood of low levels of potassium, it is recommended that you include potassium-rich foods in your diet, such as tomatoes, bananas, and citrus fruit.

Although you may experience mild diarrhea or an upset stomach, loss of appetite, dizziness, or sensitivity to sunlight (sunburn), these symptoms should cease as soon as your body adjusts to the medication. If you are taking only one dose each day, it is recommended that it be taken in the morning, preferably after breakfast. If you are taking more than one dose, take the last one approximately four to six hours before your bedtime. If you miss a dose, take it as soon as possible. However, if the next scheduled dose is within four hours, do not take the missed dose. At no time should you double up a dose.

Pregnancy
Category D (see page 103). Since the drug appears in breast milk, consult your doctor before you begin breast-feeding.

Brand Name	*Generic Name*
LOZOL	indapamide
	(in-DAP-a-mide)

How the Drug Works
By causing the kidneys to increase the flow of urine, the body eliminates more salt and water, which reduces the volume of both blood and fluid in the tissues of the body, and thereby lowers overall blood pressure.

Purpose
Treatment of hypertension and edema associated with congestive heart failure.

Dosage
• Treatment of hypertension
Adults: Initially 2.5 mg taken orally once daily, in the morning, followed, if needed, one to four weeks by an increase of 2.5 mg taken once daily.
• Treatment of edema
Adults: Initially 2.5 mg taken orally once daily in the morning, followed, if needed, in one week by an increase of 2.5 mg.

Side Effects
Uncommon: Dizziness or light-headedness, diarrhea, headache, loss of appetite, upset stomach.

Adverse Reactions
Potassium loss (dry mouth, increased thirst, irregular heart beat, mood changes, muscle cramps, nausea, fatigue and unusual weakness, and a weak pulse).
Rare: skin rash.

Drug Interaction
Increases the effects of other antihypertensive drugs.
With digitalis, there is a risk of digitalis toxicity.
With barbiturates, alcohol, and narcotic analgesics, it may drop blood pressure to dangerously low levels.

Overdosage
If any of the following symptoms develop, a physician should be notified immediately: Extreme lethargy, depression, coma.

Comments
Lozol belongs to a class of diuretics called indolines, which are much like thiazide diuretics. Like thiazide diuretics, these drugs can be used as the first drug in treating hypertension because they are long acting (one dose should last all day) and they produce few side effects. However, Lozol can be used by people with

kidney disease or impaired renal function when thiazide diuretics cannot. These diuretics are preferred by many doctors over other diuretics, specifically "loop" diuretics, because they act more gradually on the kidneys and over a longer period of time. This means you may not have to run to the bathroom as frequently while taking them.

Notify your doctor if you suffer from diabetes or gout; or kidney, liver, or pancreatic disease; or an autoimmune disease such as lupus. Do not take other medications without your doctor's approval, including any OTC preparations for coughs, colds, hay fever and sinus problems, and medicines for appetite control.

Because the drug eliminates salt and water from your body, it may also reduce your level of potassium. Some of the more common symptoms of potassium loss are excessive thirst, dry mouth, unusual weakness, lethargy, stomach cramps, restlessness and irritability. To reduce the likelihood of low levels of potassium, it is recommended that you include potassium-rich foods in your diet, such as tomatoes, bananas, and citrus fruit.

Although you may experience mild diarrhea or an upset stomach, loss of appetite, or dizziness, these symptoms should cease as soon as your body adjusts to the medication. Drinking alcohol or exercising in hot weather may increase your dizziness. On the other hand, if you have a ringing in your ears, severe stomach cramps, or sore throat and fever, notify your doctor immediately. Your blood and urine will probably be monitored periodically, especially if you have a history of gout, to determine if the drug is effective.

It is recommended that you take the tablet in the morning, preferably after breakfast. If you miss a dose, take it as soon as possible. However, if the next scheduled dose is within four hours, do not take the missed dose. At no time should you double up on a dose.

Pregnancy

Category B (see page 103). Since the drug appears in breast milk, it is recommended to not nurse while taking this drug.

LOOP DIURETICS

Brand Name
LASIX, AGRO-
FUROSEMIDE,
MYROSEMIDE

Generic Name
furosemide
(fyoo-ROH-se-mide)

How the Drug Works

By causing the kidneys to increase the flow of urine, the body eliminates more salt and water, which reduces the volume of both blood and fluid in the tissues of the body, and thereby lowers overall blood pressure.

Purpose

Treatment of hypertension or congestive heart failure.

Dosage

• Treatment of edema

Adults: Initially 20 mg to 80 mg taken orally once daily in the morning, followed by increments of 20 mg to 40 mg up to a maximum of 600 mg per day.

• Treatment of hypertension

Adults: 40 mg taken orally twice daily, followed by increases, if needed.

Side Effects

Common: Dizziness or light-headedness, orthostatic hypotension—a sudden drop in blood pressure when a person stands up after lying down or sitting.

Uncommon: Blurred vision, sensitivity to sunlight (sunburn), stomach cramps.

Adverse Reactions

Potassium loss (dry mouth, increased thirst, irregular heart beat, mood changes, muscle cramps, nausea, fatigue and unusual weakness, and a weak pulse).

Rare: Sore throat, tarry stools, fever, unusual bleeding or bruising, yellowing of the eyes or skin, skin rash, yellow vision.

Drug Interaction
Increases the effects of other antihypertensive drugs.

With digitalis, there is a risk of digitalis toxicity.

With sedatives or MAO inhibitor drugs, blood pressure may drop to dangerously low levels.

With steroids, an increased risk of hypokalemia (low levels of potassium).

Overdosage
If any of the following symptoms develop, a physician should be notified immediately: extreme lethargy, dizziness, confusion, coma.

Comments
Lasix, first introduced in 1966, belongs to a class of diuretics called loop diuretics. These drugs are not used for routine treatment of uncomplicated hypertension but rather when someone has kidney disease. Unlike thiazide diuretics, loop diuretics work quickly, which may cause you to pass large amounts of urine within a few hours of taking the drug.

Notify your doctor if you suffer from diabetes or gout; or liver, kidney, or pancreatic disease; or an autoimmune disease such as lupus. Your blood and urine will probably be monitored periodically, especially if you have a history of gout or diabetes, to determine if the drug is effective.

As the drug eliminates salt and water from your body, it may also reduce your level of potassium. Some of the more common symptoms of potassium loss are excessive thirst, dry mouth, unusual weakness, lethargy, stomach cramps, restlessness and irritability. To reduce the likelihood of low levels of potassium, it is recommended that you include potassium-rich foods in your diet, such as tomatoes, bananas, and citrus fruit.

Although you may experience mild diarrhea or an upset stomach, loss of appetite, dizziness, or a sensitivity to sunlight (sunburn), these symptoms should cease as soon as your body adjusts to the medication. Drinking alcohol or exercising in hot weather may increase your dizziness. On the other hand, if you have a ringing in your ears, severe stomach cramps, or sore throat and fever, notify your doctor immediately.

If you are taking only one dose each day, it is recommended that it be taken in the morning, preferably after breakfast. If you are taking more than one dose, take the last one approximately four to six hours before your bedtime. If you miss a dose, take it as soon as possible. However, if the next scheduled dose is within four hours, do not take the missed dose. At no time should you double up on a dose.

Pregnancy
Category C (see page 103). Since the drug appears in breast milk, consult your doctor before you begin breast-feeding.

Brand Name
BUMEX

Generic Name
bumetanide
(byoo-MET-a-nide)

How the Drug Works
By causing the kidneys to increase the flow of urine, the body eliminates more salt and water, which reduces the volume of both blood and fluid in the tissues of the body, and thereby lowers overall blood pressure.

Purpose
Treatment of heart failure.

Dosage
Adults: Initially 0.5 mg to 2 mg taken orally once daily in a single dose. If ineffective, a second and third dose can be taken each day in four-hour intervals, not exceeding 10 mg daily.

Side Effects

Common: Dizziness or light-headedness, orthostatic hypotension.

Uncommon: Blurred vision, sensitivity to sunlight (sunburn), stomach cramps.

Adverse Reactions

Potassium loss (dry mouth, increased thirst, irregular heartbeat, mood changes, muscle cramps, nausea, fatigue and unusual weakness, and a weak pulse).

Rare: Sore throat, tarry stools, fever, unusual bleeding or bruising, yellowing of the eyes or skin, skin rash, yellow vision.

Drug Interaction

Increases the effects of other antihypertensive drugs.

With digitalis, there is a risk of digitalis toxicity.

With steroids, it increases risk of hypokalemia (low levels of potassium).

Overdosage

If any of the following symptoms develop, a physician should be notified immediately: Extreme lethargy, dizziness, confusion, coma.

Comments

Bumex (bumetanide), introduced in 1983, belongs to a class of diuretics called loop diuretics. These drugs are not used for routine treatment of uncomplicated hypertension but rather when someone has kidney disease. Unlike thiazide diuretics, loop diuretics work quickly, which may cause you to pass large amounts of urine within a few hours of taking the drug. However, if you are scheduled to use with this drug for more than a few days, your doctor may recommend that you take it for three to four days and then have a one- or two-day rest period before resuming its use again.

Notify your doctor if you suffer from diabetes or gout; liver, kidney, or pancreatic disease; or an autoimmune disease such as lupus. Your blood and urine will probably be monitored periodically, especially if you have a history of gout or diabetes, to determine if the drug is effective. Because the drug eliminates salt and water from your body, it may also reduce your level of potassium. Some of the more common symptoms of potassium loss are excessive thirst, dry mouth, unusual weakness, lethargy, stomach cramps, restlessness and irritability. To reduce the likelihood of low levels of potassium, it is recommended that you include potassium-rich foods in your diet, such as tomatoes, bananas, and citrus fruit.

Although you may experience mild diarrhea or an upset stomach, loss of appetite, dizziness, or a sensitivity to sunlight (sunburn), these symptoms should cease as soon as your body adjusts to the medication. Drinking alcohol or exercising in hot weather may increase your dizziness. On the other hand, if you have a ringing in your ears, severe stomach cramps, or sore throat and fever, notify your doctor immediately.

If you are taking only one dose each day, it is recommended that it be taken in the morning, preferably after breakfast. If you are taking more than one dose, take the last one approximately four to six hours before your bedtime. If you miss a dose, take it as soon as possible. However, if the next scheduled dose is within four hours, do not take the missed dose. At no time should you double a dose.

Pregnancy
Category C (see page 103).

POTASSIUM-SPARING DIURETICS

Brand Name	*Generic Name*
ALDACTONE	spironolactone
	(speer-on-o-LAK-tone)

How the Drug Works
By causing the kidneys to increase the flow of urine, the body eliminates more salt and water, which reduces the volume of both

blood and fluid in the tissues of the body, and thereby lowers overall blood pressure, but avoids adverse effect of potassium loss.

Purpose

Treatment of edema associated with congestive heart failure; essential hypertension; low blood levels of potassium (hypokalemia)— prescribed when potassium supplements are unsuitable due to stomach upset, or when patient is prone to excessive potassium loss.

Dosage

• Treatment of heart failure

Adults: Initially 25 mg to 200 mg taken orally in single or divided doses daily.

Children: Initially 3.3 mg daily in single or divided doses.

• Treatment of essential hypertension

Adults: 50 mg to 100 mg (taken orally) twice daily, followed by increases or decreases as needed.

• Treatment of hypokalemia

Adults: 25 mg to 100 mg taken orally daily.

• Treatment of primary hyperaldosteronism

Adults: 100 mg to 400 mg daily for four days to four weeks, depending upon need.

Side Effects

Common: Nausea, dry mouth, muscle cramps, diarrhea, vomiting, sweating.

Uncommon: Breast tenderness in females, and breast enlargement in males if taken in large doses over time; deepening of voice in females; increased hair growth in females; irregular menstrual periods; decreased sexual ability in males.

Adverse Reactions

Rare: Shortness of breath; skin rash, itching; excessive potassium retention (confusion, irregular heartbeat, difficulty breathing, unusual weakness, heavy legs).

Drug Interaction
Increases the effects of other antihypertensive drugs.
Decreases the effects of oral anticoagulants.
With triamterene, may cause excessive potassium retention.

Overdosage
If any of the following symptoms develop, notify your physician immediately: Extreme lethargy, irregular heartbeats.

Comments
Aldactone (spironolactone), first introduced in 1962, belongs to a class of diuretics called potassium-sparing diuretics. Although Aldactone and other potassium-sparing diuretics are less potent than thiazide or loop diuretics (their antihypertensive effects may not begin for the first two or three days of use and maximum benefits may take up to two weeks), they are considered effective and safe in instances when potassium loss poses a problem with the other types of diuretics.

Notify your doctor if you suffer from diabetes, or liver, kidney, or heart disease. Since the drug protects from excessive potassium loss, there is no need to include potassium-rich foods in your diet, such as tomatoes, bananas, and citrus fruit, as you might when taking thiazide or loop diuretics. Avoid any potassium-containing salt substitutes as well.

Although some men may experience a distressing enlargement or tenderness of their breasts while using the drug, these symptoms disappear and the breasts usually return to normal size shortly after the drug is discontinued. If you are taking only one dose each day, it is recommended that it be taken in the morning, preferably after breakfast. To avoid stomach upset, take other doses with meals or milk. If you are taking more than one dose, take the last one approximately four to six hours before your bedtime. If you miss a dose, take it as soon as possible. However, if the next scheduled dose is within four hours, do not take the missed dose. At no time should you double up a dose.

Notify your doctor if you experience menstrual irregularities, diarrhea, stomach cramping, or skin rash. Use precaution while driving or using machinery that requires alertness or good coordination, as the drug can cause episodes of drowsiness, a lack of coordination, and mental confusion.

Pregnancy
Category D (see page 103) Since the drug appears in breast milk, consult your doctor before you begin breast-feeding.

Brand Name	*Generic Name*
MIDAMOR	amiloride hydrochloride
	(a-MIL-o-ride
	hy-dro-KLO-ride)

How the Drug Works
By causing the kidneys to increase the flow of urine, the body eliminates more salt and water, which reduces the volume of both blood and fluid in the tissues of the body, and thereby lowers overall blood pressure, but avoids the adverse effect of potassium loss.

Purpose
Treatment of hypertension congestive heart failure.

Dosage
Adults: Initially 5 mg taken orally daily; followed, if necessary, by dosage increase to 10 mg; maximum dosage is 20 mg daily.

Side Effects
Common: Headache, dry mouth, diarrhea, vomiting.
Uncommon: Nausea, muscle cramps, constipation, decreased sexual ability.

Adverse Reactions

Rare: Shortness of breath; skin rash, itching; excessive potassium retention causing confusion, irregular heartbeat, difficulty breathing, unusual weakness, heavy legs.

Drug Interaction
None significant.

Overdosage

If any of the following symptoms develop, notify your physician immediately: Extreme lethargy, irregular heartbeats, excessive drop in blood pressure.

Comments

Midamor (amiloride hydrochloride) belongs to a class of diuretics called potassium-sparing diuretics. Although Midamor and other potassium-sparing diuretics are less potent than thiazide or loop diuretics (their antihypertensive effects may not begin for the first two or three days of use and maximum benefits may take up to two weeks), they are considered effective and safe in instances when potassium loss poses a problem with the use of the other types of diuretics.

Notify your doctor if you suffer from diabetes, or liver, kidney or heart disease. Since the drug protects from excessive potassium loss, there is no need to include potassium-rich foods in your diet, such as tomatoes, bananas, and citrus fruit, as you might when taking thiazide or loop diuretics. Avoid any potassium-containing salt substitutes as well.

If you are taking only one dose a day, it is recommended that it be taken in the morning, preferably after breakfast. To avoid stomach upset, take other doses with meals or milk. If you are taking more than one dose, take the last one approximately four to six hours before your bedtime. If you miss a dose, take it as soon as possible. However, if the next scheduled dose is within four hours, do not take the missed dose. At no time should you double a dose.

Notify your doctor if you experience muscle weakness, fatigue, or muscle cramps. Use precaution while driving or using machinery that requires alertness or good coordination, as the drug can cause episodes of blurred vision, headaches, or dizziness.

Pregnancy
Category B (see page 103).

Brand Name	Generic Name
DYRENIUM	triamterene
	(try-AM-te-reen)

How the Drug Works
By causing the kidneys to increase the flow of urine, the body eliminates more salt and water, which reduces the volume of both blood and fluid in the tissues of the body, and thereby lowers overall blood pressure, but avoids the adverse effect of potassium loss.

Purpose
Treatment of congestive heart failure.

Dosage
Adults: Initially 100 mg taken orally twice daily after meals, followed, if necessary, by dosages up to 300 mg daily.

Side Effects
Common: Dizziness, headaches, dry mouth, diarrhea, vomiting.
Uncommon: Nausea, muscle cramps, constipation.

Adverse Reactions
Fever, sore throat, mouth sores, unusual bleeding or bruising.

Drug Interaction
None significant.

Overdosage
If any of the following symptoms develop, notify your physician immediately: Extreme lethargy, excessive drop in blood pressure.

Comments
Dyrenium, introduced in 1964, belongs to a class of diuretics called potassium-sparing diuretics. Although Dyrenium and other potassium-sparing diuretics are less potent than thiazide or loop diuretics (their antihypertensive effects may not begin for the first two or three days of use and maximum benefits may take up to two weeks), they are considered effective and safe in instances when potassium loss poses a problem with the use of the other types of diuretics.

Notify your doctor if you suffer from diabetes, or liver, kidney, or heart disease. Since the drug protects from excessive potassium loss, there is no need to include potassium-rich foods in your diet, such as tomatoes, bananas, and citrus fruit, as you might when taking thiazide or loop diuretics. Avoid any potassium-containing salt substitutes as well.

If you are taking only one dose each day, it is recommended that it be taken in the morning, preferably after breakfast. To avoid stomach upset, take other doses with meals or milk. If you are taking more than one dose, take the last one approximately four to six hours before your bedtime. If you miss a dose, take it as soon as possible. However, if the next scheduled dose is within four hours, do not take the missed dose. At no time should you double up a dose.

Notify your doctor if you experience fever or sore throat or signs of unusual bruising or bleeding. Limited exposure to sunlight may lead to sunburn, as one of the drug's side effects is photosensitivity.

Pregnancy
Category D (see page 103). Since the drug appears in breast milk, consult your doctor before you begin breast-feeding.

DIURETIC COMBINATIONS

Brand Name
DYAZIDE

Generic Name
triamterene and
hydrochlorothiazide
(try-AM-te-reen and
hy-dro-KLO-ro-thy-
a-zide)

How the Drug Works
By causing the kidneys to increase the flow of urine, the body eliminates more salt and water (without risk of excessive potassium loss) which reduces the volume of both blood and fluid in the tissues of the body, and thereby lowers overall blood pressure.

Purpose
Treatment of edema associated with congestive heart failure and hypertension.

Dosage
Adults: One capsule (with fixed amounts of 50 mg triamterene and 25 mg hydrochlorothiazide) twice a day, increased to a maximum of four capsules daily. Some patients may require only one capsule a day or one every other day.

Side Effects
Common: Nausea, loss of appetite, stomach cramps, diarrhea, vomiting.
Uncommon: Dizziness or light-headedness, sensitivity to sunlight (sunburn), decreased sexual ability, headaches, constipation.

Adverse Reactions
Rare: Sore throat; skin rash; joint pain; fever; unusual bleeding or bruising; yellowish skin; red or painful, burning tongue; cracked corners of mouth.

Drug Interaction
Increases the effects of other antihypertensive drugs.
Decreases the effects of oral anticoagulants.
With spironolactone, may cause excessive potassium retention.

Overdosage
If any of the following symptoms develop, notify your physician immediately: Extreme lethargy, unusual thirst, irregular heartbeats.

Comments
Dyazide, first introduced in 1964, belongs to a class of diuretics called diuretic combinations and is composed of triamterene, which conserves the body's potassium, and hydrochlorothiazide. It is a mild diuretic that poses little risk of potassium loss and is used as a "Step 1" (see page 46) medication in the treatment of mild or moderate hypertension. In the treatment of edema, the drug may be needed for two or three days; in the treatment of hypertension, the drug may be used for as long as two or three weeks.

Notify your doctor if you suffer from diabetes, or liver, kidney, or heart disease. Since the drug protects from excessive potassium loss, there is no need to include potassium-rich foods in your diet, such as tomatoes, bananas, and citrus fruit, as you might when taking thiazide or loop diuretics. Avoid any potassium-containing salt substitutes as well.

If you are taking only one dose each day, it is recommended that it be taken in the morning, preferably after breakfast. To avoid stomach upset, take other doses with meals or milk. If you are taking more than one dose, take the last one approximately four to six hours before your bedtime. If you miss a dose, take it as soon as possible. However, if the next scheduled dose is within four hours, do not take the missed dose. At no time should you double a dose.

Pregnancy
Safety for use during pregnancy has not been formally established. However, since the drug contains hydrochlorothiazide,

it is recommended that this drug be treated as Category D (see page 103). Since the drug appears in breast milk, consult your doctor before you begin breast-feeding.

Brand Name
MAXZIDE

Generic Name
Triamterene and Hydrochlorothiazide (try-AM-te-reen and hy-dro-KLO-ro-THY-a-zide)

Comments

Maxzide, which also belongs to a class of diuretics called diuretic combinations, is very similar to Dyazide (page 140), although more potent. Its usual dosage is one tab (75 mg triamterene and 50 mg hydrochlorothiazide) daily and is used primarily in cases where someone who requires a thiazide diuretic suffers from calcium loss from another medication or has a history of arrhythmia. Its side effects, potential adverse reactions, and drug interactions resemble those of Dyazide.

Pregnancy

Category C (see page 103).

Brand Name
MODURETIC

Generic Name
amiloride hydrochloride and hydrochlorothiazide (a-MIL-o-ride hy-dro-KLO-ride and hy-dro-klo-ro-THY-a-zide)

How the Drug Works

By causing the kidneys to increase the flow of urine, the body eliminates more salt and water, which reduces the volume of both blood and fluid in the tissues of the body, and thereby lowers overall blood pressure, while avoiding risk of excessive potassium or calcium loss.

Purpose

Treatment of hypertension; congestive heart failure.

Dosage

Adults: Initially one tab (5 mg amiloride hydrochloride and 50 mg hydrochlorothiazide) daily, and if needed, followed by two tabs daily in single or divided doses.

Side Effects

Common: Nausea, loss of appetite, stomach cramps, diarrhea, vomiting.

Uncommon: Dizziness or light-headedness, sensitivity to sunlight (sunburn), decreased sexual ability, headaches, constipation.

Adverse Reactions

Rare: Sore throat; skin rash; joint pain; fever; unusual bleeding or bruising; yellowish skin; red or painful, burning tongue; cracked corners of mouth.

Drug Interaction

Increases the effects of other antihypertensive drugs.

Decreases the effects of oral anticoagulants.

With spironolactone, may cause excessive potassium retention.

Overdosage

If any of the following symptoms develop, notify your physician immediately: Extreme lethargy, unusual thirst, irregular heartbeats.

Comments

Moduretic, first introduced in 1964, belongs to a class of diuretics called diuretic combinations. This drug—composed of amiloride, which conserves the body's potassium, and hydrochlorothiazide—is a mild diuretic that poses little risk of potassium or calcium loss and is used as a "Step 1" medication in the treatment of mild or moderate hypertension. In the treatment of edema, the drug may be needed for two or three days; in the treatment of hypertension, the drug may be used for as long as two or three weeks.

Notify your doctor if you suffer from diabetes, or liver, kidney, or heart disease. Since the drug protects from excessive potassium loss, there is no need to include potassium-rich foods in your diet, such as tomatoes, bananas, and citrus fruit, as you might when taking thiazide or loop diuretics. Avoid any potassium-containing salt substitutes as well.

If you are taking only one dose each day, it is recommended that it be taken in the morning, preferably after breakfast. To avoid stomach upset, take other doses with meals or milk. If you are taking more than one dose, take the last one approximately four to six hours before your bedtime. If you miss a dose, take it as soon as possible. However, if the next scheduled dose is within four hours, do not take the missed dose. At no time should you double a dose.

Pregnancy

Category B (see page 103).

SEVEN
Beta Blockers

B1-SELECTIVE BETA-ADRENERGIC BLOCKERS

Brand Name	*Generic Name*
LOPRESSOR	metoprolol
TENORMIN	atenolol

NONSELECTIVE BETA-ADRENERGIC BLOCKERS

Brand Name	*Generic Name*
BLOCADREN	timolol maleate
INDERAL, INDERAL LA	propranolol hydrochloride
SECTRAL	acebutolol hydrochloride
CORGARD	nadolol
VISKEN	pindolol
LEVATOL	penbutolol
CARTROL	carteolol hydrochloride
KERLONE	betaxolol

ALPHA- AND BETA-ADRENERGIC BLOCKERS

Brand Name	*Generic Name*
NORMODYNE, TRANDATE	labetalol hydrochloride

Beta blockers block the passage of stimulating substances to beta receptors in the body. These receptors are found at various sites in the body, primarily in the brain, the lungs, around the eyes, and in the heart muscle. When the heart is exposed to less of the body's natural stimulating substances, such as epinephrine, its work load is reduced and blood pressure is lowered. This makes beta blockers effective in the treatment of high blood pressure and hypertension, and they are generally described as "antihypertensives."

There are two types of beta receptor: beta-1, located in the heart muscle, and beta-2, located in the lungs and blood vessels. Some beta blockers, called B1-selective drugs, affect primarily the heart, while other beta blockers, nonselective, affect not only the heart but the lungs and the blood vessels. Some people, such those suffering from asthma, may not tolerate beta blockers that affect the beta-2 receptor site in the lungs.

Beta blockers are also used to treat angina and arrhythmia and are prescribed to prevent migraine headaches, treat glaucoma, and reduce situational anxiety (stage fright).

Potential risks: Beta blockers have various side effects; some can cause depression and some aggravate congestive heart failure by slowing the heartbeat more than others. Alpha- and some beta-adrenergic blockers, such as Normodyne and Trandate, should not be used by patients with a history of any respiratory diseases, as they affect the lungs more than B1-selective beta blockers; but all beta blockers should be used cautiously if you have poor circulation or a history of heart failure. People with diabetes should also be made aware of the fact that the action of these drugs may suppress the normal warning signs of a diabetic attack, such as tremors or heart palpitations.

If you are taking beta blockers, ask your doctor about any exercise regimen you want to undertake or continue, since beta blockers can reduce the effectiveness of the heart to perform at optimal levels. Because of their direct effect on the heart, beta blockers should not be suddenly discontinued, especially after you have been taking them for several months, since the abrupt

146

change could produce immediate and severe recurrence of your original symptoms.

A wide range of these drugs is available, so your doctor has several choices if the one you are taking should cause an unacceptable side effect or adverse reaction.

B1-SELECTIVE BETA-ADRENERGIC BLOCKERS

Brand Name	*Generic Name*
LOPRESSOR	metoprolol
	(me-TOH-pro-lol)

How the Drug Works

By blocking actions of the sympathetic nervous system: It slows the heart rate and reduces tension in the walls of the blood vessels. Reduces blood pressure levels.

Purpose

Hypertension; angina pectoris; acute myocardial infarction.

Dosage

• Hypertension

Adults: Initially 50 mg (taken orally) daily in single or divided doses, followed by increases at minimum intervals of seven days if needed, up to a maximum dosage of 450 mg daily.

• Angina pectoris

Adults: Initially 50 mg taken orally in two divided doses, followed by increases at minimum intervals of seven days if needed, up to a maximum dosage of 400 mg daily.

• Acute Myocardial Infarction

Adults: Initially 5 mg intravenously every two minutes up to a total of 15 mg followed by oral maintenance.

Side Effects
Common: Dizziness or light-headedness, diarrhea, fatigue.
Uncommon: Anxiety, headache, nausea, vivid dreams, itching and rash.

Adverse Reactions
Fatigue, slow heartbeat, wheezing, depression, hallucinations, cold hands and feet, dry mouth, heartburn, constipation, heart palpitations. It also masks the effects of low blood pressure.

Drug Interaction
Increases the effects of other hypertensive drugs, sedatives, tranquilizers, digitalis preparations, phenothiazine, reserpine, and calcium antagonists.

Overdosage
If any of the following symptoms develop, notify your physician immediately: Slow heartbeat, severe dizziness or fainting, difficulty breathing.

Comments
Introduced in this country in 1978, Lopressor is considered a B1-selective beta-adrenergic blocker, which means that this beta-blocker drug affects primarily the receptor sites in the heart ("cardioselective") at doses less than 200 mg, whereas nonselective beta blockers such as Blocadren and Inderal affect the receptor sites in the lungs and the blood vessels as well. Hence, this beta blocker is less likely to produce wheezing or breathing difficulties.

Lopressor (and Tenormin) offer an advantage to diabetic patients, as they do not delay recovery from hypoglycemia as do the nonselective beta blockers. These drugs should be taken at the same time each day. In addition to using it in the treatment of high blood pressure, angina, and to give long-term protection following acute myocardial infarction (heart attack), doctors use it to treat irregular heartbeats and to prevent migraines and tremors. Doctors have also found Lopressor helpful in the treatment of aggressive behaviors.

Notify your doctor if you have been taking monoamine oxidase (MAO) inhibitor during the past 14 days; if you suffer from asthma, allergic rhinitis (hay fever), or congestive heart failure; or if your heartbeat is below 50 beats per minute. Patients taking insulin, who have fluctuations in the blood sugar, must be closely watched since they may develop dangerously low sugar levels in the absence of their usual warning symptoms of rapid heartbeat and sweating. Your blood pressure will probably be closely monitored for the first four weeks to determine if the drug is effective.

You should not take any OTC medication, such as nasal decongestants or cold preparations, unless you check with your doctor or pharmacist first, since many B1-selective beta-adrenergic blockers can cause a rise in your blood pressure. If you miss a dose, take it as soon as possible. However, if the next scheduled dose is within four hours, do not take the missed dose. At no time should you take a double dose. When preparing to discontinue its use, do not stop abruptly, as that may aggravate the angina or increase risk of a heart attack; reduce its dosage over a one- to two-week period. Use precaution while driving or using machinery that requires alertness or good coordination.

Avoid excessive salt in your diet and take the drug about an hour before eating. While you are taking this drug, exercise or heavy exertion may cause light-headedness. If your heart is prevented from increasing its rate commensurate with your level of activity, your doctor should be consulted to recommend for you an exercise target heart rate. And if you are to take a stress test, consult your doctor whether to taper or reduce the level of your medication. Smoking, which is strongly discouraged, can be especially harmful because it can increase the constriction of the lung's bronchial tubes and induce wheezing.

If you take a beta blocker, you should ask your doctor to teach you how to take your pulse, so you can monitor your heart rate before taking a medicine that might lower your rate too much and cause symptoms of fatigue or dizziness. Additionally, if you have palpitations (sensation of your heart throbbing) you can document the heart rate and rhythm, which helps your doctor make the right diagnosis. It's important that you notify your doctor immediately if you become pregnant when taking a beta blocker.

Pregnancy
Category C (see page 103).

Brand Name	*Generic Name*
TENORMIN	atenolol (a-TEN-a-lol)

How the Drug Works
By blocking actions of the sympathetic nervous system, it slows the heart rate and reduces tension in the walls of the blood vessels, thereby reducing blood pressure levels.

Purpose
Treatment of hypertension and angina pectoris.

Dosage
• Hypertension
Adults: Initially 50 mg taken orally once daily, followed if needed by increases every two weeks of 100 mg a day.
• Angina pectoris
Adults: Initially 50 mg taken orally once daily, followed if needed by increases of 100 mg once daily; maximum dosage is 200 mg once daily.

Side Effects
Common: Dizziness or light-headedness, insomnia, decreased sexual ability, fatigue.

Uncommon: Anxiety, dry eyes, constipation, headache, nausea, vivid dreams, itching and rash, stuffy nose.

Adverse Reactions

Extreme fatigue, slow heartbeat, wheezing, depression, hallucinations, cold hands and feet, dry mouth, heartburn, constipation, heart palpitations. It also masks the effects of low blood sugar.

Drug Interaction

Increases the effects of other hypertensive drugs, sedatives, tranquilizers, digitalis preparations, phenothiazine, reserpine, and calcium antagonists.

Overdosage

If any of the following symptoms develop, notify your physician immediately: Slow heartbeat, severe dizziness or fainting, difficulty breathing.

Comments

Introduced in this country in 1973, Tenormin is considered a B1-selective beta-adrenergic blocker, which means that this beta-blocker drug affects primarily the receptor sites in the heart ("cardioselective") at doses of 100 mg or less, whereas nonselective beta blockers such as Blocadren and Inderal affect the receptor sites in the lungs and the blood vessels as well. Hence, this beta blocker is less likely to produce wheezing or breathing difficulties.

Tenormin (and Lopressor) offer an advantage to diabetic patients as they do not delay recovery from hypoglycemia as do the nonselective beta blockers. Doctors use Tenormin not only for the treatment of high blood pressure and angina, but also to treat irregular heartbeats and to prevent migraines, tremors, and situational anxiety (stage fright).

Notify your doctor if you have been taking monoamine oxidase (MAO) inhibitor during the past 14 days; if you suffer from asthma, allergic rhinitis (hay fever), or congestive heart failure;

or if your heartbeat is below 50 beats per minute. Your blood pressure will probably be closely monitored for the first four weeks to determine if the drug is effective.

You should not take any OTC medication such as nasal decongestants or cold preparations, unless you check with your doctor or pharmacist first, since many of these drugs can cause a rise in your blood pressure. If you miss a dose, take it as soon as possible. However, if the next scheduled dose is within four hours, do not take the missed dose. At no time should you take a double dose. When preparing to discontinue Tenormin's use, do not stop abruptly, as it may aggravate the angina or increase risk of a heart attack; reduce its dosage over a one- to two-week period. Use precaution while driving or using machinery that requires alertness or good coordination.

Avoid excessive salt in your diet and take Tenormin about an hour before eating. While taking Tenormin, exercise or heavy exertion may cause light-headedness. If your heart is prevented from increasing its rate commensurate with your level of activity, your doctor should be consulted to recommend an exercise target heart rate for you. If you are to take a stress test, consult your doctor whether to reduce your medication. Smoking, which is strongly discouraged, can be especially harmful because it can increase the constriction of the lung's bronchial tubes and induce wheezing.

If you take a beta blocker you should ask your doctor to teach you how to take your pulse. You then can monitor your heart rate before taking a medicine that could lower your rate too much and cause symptoms of fatigue or dizziness. Additionally, if you have palpitations (sensation of your heart throbbing) you can document the heart rate and rhythm, which helps your doctor make the right diagnosis. It is important that you notify your doctor immediately if you become pregnant when taking a beta blocker.

Pregnancy:
Category C (see page 103).

NONSELECTIVE BETA-ADRENERGIC BLOCKERS

Brand Name
BLOCADREN

Generic Name
timolol maleate (TIM-o-lol MAL-ee-ayt)

How the Drug Works

By blocking actions of the sympathetic nervous system, it slows the heart rate, reduces tension in the walls of the blood vessels, and restricts the release by the kidneys of an enzyme called renin, thereby reducing blood pressure levels.

Purpose

Treatment of hypertension (high blood pressure), and to provide long-term protection following acute myocardial infarction (heart attack).

Dosage

• Hypertension
Adults: Initially 10 mg taken orally twice daily, followed by an increase up to 60 mg daily in divided doses. Usual daily dosage is 20 mg to 40 mg, in divided doses.
• Following a myocardial infarction
Adults: 10 mg taken orally twice daily.

Side Effects

Common: Dizziness or light-headedness, trouble sleeping, fatigue.
Uncommon: Anxiety, constipation, diarrhea, headache, nausea, itching of the skin, vivid dreams, leg cramps, cold fingers and toes upon exposure to cold weather, decreased libido (sexual drive).

Adverse Reactions

Constant fatigue, slow heartbeat, wheezing (patients with history of asthma or emphysema), depression, skin rash, hallucinations, confusion (in elderly). It also masks the effects of low blood sugar.

Rare: Fever and sore throat, chest pains, back pain, unusual bleeding or bruising.

Drug Interaction

Increases the effects of other hypertensive drugs, sedatives, tranquilizers, digitalis preparations, and calcium antagonists.

Response to hypoglycemia (low blood sugar) is blunted (see "Comments" below).

Overdosage

If any of the following symptoms develop, a physician should be notified immediately: Slow heartbeat (bradycardia), severe dizziness or fainting, difficulty breathing, seizures.

Comments

Blocadren, introduced in 1972, is frequently used in the treatment of essential hypertension and was the first beta blocker generally used to treat patients recovering from a myocardial infarction. Doctors also use this drug to treat irregular heartbeats and in the prevention of migraines.

Notify your doctor if you have been taking a monoamine oxidase (MAO) inhibitor drug in the past 14 days; suffer from diabetes mellitus, asthma, allergic rhinitis (hay fever), or congestive heart failure; or if your heart rate is below 50 beats per minute. Your blood pressure will probably be closely monitored for the first four weeks to determine if the drug is effective.

Patients taking insulin, who have fluctuations in their blood sugar, must be closely watched, since they may develop dangerously low sugar levels in the absence of their usual warning symptoms of rapid heartbeat and sweating.

You should not take any OTC medication, such as nasal decongestants or cold preparations, unless you check with your doctor or pharmacist first, since many of these drugs can cause a rise in your blood pressure. Never increase the dosage of your medication without a doctor's approval. If you miss a dose, take it as soon as possible. However, if the next scheduled dose is within four hours, do not take the missed dose. At no time should you take a double dose. It is very important to understand that when preparing to discontinue its use, *do not stop abruptly*, as this may aggravate the angina or increase risk of a heart attack; reduce its dosage over a one- to two-week period. Use precaution while driving or using machinery that requires alertness or good coordination.

Avoid excessive salt in your diet and take Blocadren about an hour before eating. While you are taking this drug, exercise or heavy exertion may cause light-headedness. If your heart is prevented from increasing its rate commensurate with your level of activity, your doctor should be consulted to recommend an exercise target heart rate for you. If you are to take a stress test, consult your doctor whether to reduce your medication. Smoking, which is strongly discouraged, can be especially harmful because it can increase the constriction of the lung's bronchial tubes and induce wheezing.

If you take a beta blocker, you should ask your doctor to teach you how to take your pulse. You then can monitor your heart rate before taking a medicine that can lower your rate too much and cause symptoms of fatigue or dizziness. Additionally, if you have palpitations (sensation of your heart throbbing) you can document the heart rate and rhythm, which helps your doctor make the right diagnosis. It is important that you notify your doctor immediately if you become pregnant when taking a beta blocker.

Pregnancy
Category C (see page 103).

Brand Name	Generic Name
INDERAL, INDERAL LA	propranolol hydrochloride (pro-PRAN-o-lol hy-dro-KLO-ride)

How the Drug Works

By blocking actions of the sympathetic nervous system, it slows the heart rate, reduces tension in the walls of the blood vessels, and restricts the release by the kidneys of an enzyme called renin, thereby reducing blood pressure levels.

Purpose

Treatment of essential hypertension, angina pectoris, cardiac arrhythmias, acute myocardial infarction, migraine headaches, symptoms of mitral valve prolapse.

Dosage

• Essential hypertension

Adults: Initially 40 mg taken orally daily in divided doses, followed by gradual increases at three- to seven-day intervals if needed up to a maximum dosage of 640 mg daily. The usual maintenance dosage is 120 mg to 240 mg daily. Inderal LA (long acting) can be taken once daily because of its longer duration of action.

Children: Initially 0.5 mg taken orally daily in divided doses, followed by increments up to 16 mg daily; the usual maintenance dosage is 1 mg to 2 mg daily.

• Long-term management of cardiac arrhythmias

Adults: 10 mg to 30 mg (taken orally) three or four times daily before meals and at bedtime.

• Treatment of angina pectoris:

Adults: Tablets—80 mg to 320 mg taken orally two to four times daily. LA capsules—80 mg (taken orally) once daily, and in increments every three to seven days, if necessary, to 320 mg.

• Following acute myocardial infarction:

Adults: Tablets—180 mg to 240 mg taken orally two or three times daily.

Side Effects

Common: Dizziness or light-headedness, trouble sleeping, fatigue.

Uncommon: Anxiety, constipation, diarrhea, headache, nausea, itching of the skin, vivid dreams, cool fingers and toes.

Adverse Reactions

Constant fatigue, slow heartbeat, wheezing (patients with history of asthma or emphysema), depression, skin rash, hallucinations, confusion (in elderly). (The drugs also mask the effects of low blood sugar.)

Rare: Fever, chest pains, back pain, unusual bleeding or bruising.

Drug Interaction

Increases the effects of other hypertensive drugs, sedatives, tranquilizers, digitalis preparations.

Overdosage

If any of the following symptoms develop, a physician should be notified immediately: Slow heartbeat, severe dizziness or fainting, difficulty breathing, seizures.

Comments

Inderal (propranolol), introduced in 1965, is frequently a first drug used in the treatment of essential hypertension. Of all the beta-adrenergic blocking drugs, propranolol may have the greatest number of uses. In addition to using it in the treatment of high blood pressure, angina, irregular heartbeat, and long-term protection following acute myocardial infarction (heart attack), doctors use it to treat the symptoms of hypertrophic cardiomyopathy, to correct irregular heartbeats, and to prevent migraines and tremors. Moreover, doctors have found Inderal helpful in the treatment of rage, situational anxiety (stage fright), recurrent gastrointestinal bleeding, schizophrenia, acute pain, and the symptoms associated with alcohol withdrawal, among other conditions.

Notify your doctor if you have been taking a monoamine oxidase (MAO) inhibitor drug in the past 14 days; if you suffer from diabetes mellitus, asthma, allergic rhinitis (hay fever), emphysema, or congestive heart failure; or if your heart rate is below 50 beats per minute. Patients taking insulin, who have fluctuations in the blood sugar, must be closely watched since they may develop dangerously low sugar levels in the absence of the usual warning symptoms of rapid heartbeat and sweating. Your blood pressure will probably be closely monitored for the first four weeks to determine if the drug is effective.

You should not take any OTC medication, such as nasal decongestants or cold preparations, unless you check with your doctor or pharmacist first, since many of these drugs can cause a rise in your blood pressure. Never increase the dosage of your medication without a doctor's approval. If you miss a dose, take it as soon as possible. However, if the next scheduled dose is within four hours, do not take the missed dose. At no time should you take a double dose. When preparing to discontinue Inderal, do not stop abruptly, as it may aggravate the angina or increase risk of a heart attack; reduce the dosage over a one- to two-week period. Use precaution while driving or using machinery that requires alertness or good coordination.

Avoid excessive salt in your diet and take Inderal about an hour before eating. While you are taking Inderal, exercise or heavy exertion may cause light-headedness. If your heart is prevented from increasing its rate commensurate with your level of activity, your doctor should be consulted to recommend an exercise target heart rate for you. If you are to take a stress test, consult your doctor whether to reduce your medication. Smoking, which is strongly discouraged, can be especially harmful because it can increase the constriction of the lung's bronchial tubes and induce wheezing.

If you take a beta blocker, you should ask your doctor to teach you how to take your pulse. You then can monitor your heart rate before taking a medicine that could lower your rate too much and cause symptoms of fatigue or dizziness. In addition, if you have palpitations (sensation of your heart throbbing) you can document the heart rate and rhythm, which helps your doctor make the right diagnosis. It is important that you notify your doctor immediately if you become pregnant when taking a beta blocker.

Pregnancy
Category C (see page 103).

Brand Name	*Generic Name*
SECTRAL	acebutolol hydrochloride (as-e-BYOO-to-lol hydro-KLO-ride)

How the Drug Works
By blocking actions of the sympathetic nervous system, it slows the heart rate, reduces tension in the walls of the blood vessels, and restricts the release by the kidneys of an enzyme called renin, thereby reducing blood pressure levels.

Purpose
Treatment of hypertension and premature ventricular contractions (ventricular arrhythmia).

Dosage
• Essential hypertension
Adults: Initially 200 to 400 mg taken orally daily in a single dose (in rare cases, in divided doses). Maintenance dose is 400 mg to 800 mg daily, but in instances of severe hypertension, given with another antihypertensive such as a thiazide diuretic, a maximum of 1,200 mg per day in two divided doses.
• Ventricular arrhythmia
Adults: Initially 200 mg daily in divided doses, then increase as needed; maintenance doses are 600 mg to 1,200 mg daily.

Side Effects
Common: Fatigue, headaches, dizziness or light-headedness, trouble sleeping.

Uncommon: Anxiety, constipation, stomachaches, diarrhea, headache, depression, urinary hesitancies, nausea, itching of the skin, weight gain, vivid dreams, nervousness, edema, decreased sexual ability, cool fingers and toes.

Adverse Reactions

Constant fatigue, slow heartbeat, wheezing (patients with history of asthma or emphysema), dyspnea, skin rash, palpitations, chest pains, back pain, joint pain, burning of the eyes. It also masks the effects of low blood sugar.

Drug Interaction

Increases the effects of other hypertensive drugs, sedatives, tranquilizers, digitalis preparations, and calcium antagonists.

Response to hypoglycemia (low blood sugar) is blunted.

Overdosage

If any of the following symptoms develop, notify your physician immediately: Excessive bradycardia (slow heartbeat), severe congestive heart failure, seizures, low blood pressure.

Comments

Sectral (acebutolol) is used to treat high blood pressure and irregular heartbeats. As a cardioselective drug it is relatively selective for B1 receptors and therefore produces fewer bronchospasms than nonselective beta blockers, which also affect B2 receptors in the lungs.

Notify your doctor if you have been taking a monoamine oxidase (MAO) inhibitor drug in the past 14 days; if you suffer from diabetes mellitus, asthma, allergic rhinitis (hay fever), emphysema, congestive heart failure, or kidney disease; or if your pulse rate is below 50 beats per minute. Patients taking insulin, who have fluctuations in the blood sugar, must be closely watched since they may develop dangerously low sugar levels in the absence of the usual warning symptoms of rapid heartbeat and sweating. Your blood pressure will probably be closely monitored for the first four weeks to determine if the drug is effective.

You should not take any OTC medication, such as nasal decongestants or cold preparations, unless you check with your doctor or pharmacist first, since many of these drugs can cause a rise in your blood pressure. Never increase the dosage of your medication without a doctor's approval. If you miss a dose, take it as soon as possible. However, if the next scheduled dose is within four hours, do not take the missed dose. At no time should you double a dose. When preparing to discontinue its use, do not stop abruptly, as it may aggravate the angina or increase risk of a heart attack; reduce its dosage over a one- to two-week period. Use precaution while driving or using machinery that requires alertness or good coordination.

This drug can be taken with meals, if that's convenient. While taking this drug, exercise or heavy exertion may cause lightheadedness. If your heart is prevented from increasing its rate commensurate with your level of activity, your doctor should be consulted to recommend an exercise target heart rate for you. If you are to take a stress test, consult your doctor whether to reduce your medication. Smoking, which is strongly discouraged, can be especially harmful because it can increase the constriction of the lung's bronchial tubes and induce wheezing.

If you take a beta blocker, you should ask your doctor to teach you how to take your pulse. You then can monitor your heart rate before taking a medicine which can lower your rate too much and cause symptoms of fatigue or dizziness. Additionally, if you have palpitations, you can document the heart rate and rhythm which helps your doctor make the right diagnosis. It is important that you notify your doctor immediately if you become pregnant when taking a beta blocker.

Pregnancy

Category B (see page 103). Since the drug appears in breast milk, nursing is not recommended while taking this drug.

Brand Name	Generic Name
CORGARD	nadolol (NAY-do-lol)

How the Drug Works

Reduces blood pressure levels by blocking actions of the sympathetic nervous system. It slows the heart rate, reduces tension in the walls of the blood vessels, and restricts the release by the kidneys of an enzyme called renin.

Purpose

Treatment of angina pectoris and hypertension.

Dosage

• Angina pectoris

Adults: Initially 40 mg taken orally daily in a single dose, followed by gradual increases of 40 mg to 80 mg daily at three- to seven-day intervals if needed up to a maximum dosage of 240 mg daily; usual maintenance dose is 40 mg to 80 mg once daily.

• Essential hypertension

Adults: Initially 40 mg taken orally with or without a diuretic in a single dose, followed by gradual increases of 40 mg to 80 mg daily at three- to seven-day intervals if needed up to a maximum dosage of 320 mg daily; usual maintenance dose is 40 mg to 80 mg once daily.

Side Effects

Common: Dizziness or light-headedness, trouble sleeping, fatigue.

Uncommon: Constipation, diarrhea, headache, nausea, dry eyes, blurred vision, cool fingers and toes.

Adverse Reactions

Slow heartbeat, wheezing (patients with history of asthma or emphysema), skin rash, slurred speech.

Rare: fever, facial swelling. It also masks the effects of low blood sugar.

Drug Interaction
Increases the effects of other hypertensive drugs, sedatives, tranquilizers, digitalis preparations, and calcium antagonists.
Response to hypoglycemia (low blood sugar) is blunted.
With epinephrine, will cause sharp rise in blood pressure.

Overdosage
If any of the following symptoms develop, a physician should be notified immediately: Excessive and rapid heartbeat, hypotension, bronchospasm, heart failure.

Comments
Corgard (nadolol), introduced in 1980, is primarily used in the treatment of coronary artery disease to prevent exercise-induced angina and essential hypertension. Like many of the other beta-adrenergic blocking drugs, nadolol has many other uses. Doctors use it to treat arrhythmia, aggressive behavior, antipsychotic (drug)-induced restlessness, situational anxiety (stage fright), and bleeding of the esophagus, and to prevent migraine headaches and reduce pressure on the eye (a hypertension symptom).

Notify your doctor if you have been taking a monoamine oxidase (MAO) inhibitor drug in the past 14 days; if you suffer from diabetes mellitus, asthma, allergic rhinitis (hay fever), emphysema, or congestive heart failure; or if your pulse rate is below 50 beats per minute. Patients taking insulin, who have fluctuations in the blood sugar, must be closely watched since they may develop dangerously low sugar levels without their usual warning symptoms of rapid heartbeat and sweating. Your blood pressure will probably be closely monitored for the first four weeks to determine if the drug is effective.

You should not take any OTC medication, such as nasal decongestants or cold preparations, unless you check with your doctor or pharmacist first since many of these drugs can cause a rise in your blood pressure. Never increase the dosage of your medication without a doctor's approval. If you miss a dose, take it as soon as possible. However, if the next scheduled dose is within four hours, do not take the missed dose. At no time should you double a dose. When preparing to discontinue its use, do not stop abruptly, as it may aggravate the angina or increase risk of a heart attack; reduce its dosage over a one- to two-week period. Use precaution while driving or using machinery that requires alertness or good coordination.

This drug can be taken with meals, if that's convenient. While taking this drug, exercise or heavy exertion may cause lightheadedness. If your heart is prevented from increasing its rate commensurate with your level of activity, your doctor should be consulted to recommend for you an exercise target heart rate. If you are to take a stress test, consult your doctor whether to taper or reduce the level of your medication. Smoking, which is strongly discouraged, can be especially harmful because it can increase the constriction of the lung's bronchial tubes and induce wheezing.

If you take a beta blocker, you should ask your doctor to teach you how to take your pulse. You then can monitor your heart rate before taking a medicine which can lower your rate too much and cause symptoms of fatigue or dizziness. Additionally, if you have palpitations (sensation of your heart throbbing) you can document the heart rate and rhythm, which helps your doctor make the right diagnosis. It is important that you notify your doctor immediately if you become pregnant when taking a beta-blocker.

Pregnancy
Category C (see page 103). Since this drug appears in breast milk, nursing is not recommended while taking it.

Brand Name	*Generic Name*
VISKEN	pindolol (PIN-do-lol)

How the Drug Works
Reduces blood pressure levels by blocking actions of the sympathetic nervous system. It slows the heart rate, reduces tension in

the walls of the blood vessels, and restricts the release by the kidneys of an enzyme called renin.

Purpose
Treatment of hypertension.

Dosage
Adults: Initially 5 mg taken orally daily in a single dose, followed by increases of 10 mg every three to four weeks if necessary up to a maximum of 60 mg daily.

Side Effects
Common: Trouble sleeping, dizziness or light-headedness, fatigue, nervousness, edema, decreased sexual ability.

Uncommon: Anxiety, constipation, stomachaches, diarrhea, headache, nausea, itching of the skin, weight gain, vivid dreams, cool fingers and toes.

Adverse Reactions
Constant fatigue; slow heartbeat; wheezing (patients with history of asthma or emphysema), dyspnea (labored breathing); skin rash; palpitations; chest pains; back pain; muscle cramps; burning sensation in the eyes. It also masks the effects of low blood sugar.

Drug Interaction
Increases the effects of other hypertensive drugs, sedatives, tranquilizers, digitalis preparations, and calcium antagonists.

With epinephrine, will cause sharp rise in blood pressure.

Overdosage
If any of the following symptoms develop, notify your physician immediately: Excessive and rapid heartbeat, low blood pressure, heart failure.

Comments
Visken (pindolol) was the first beta blocker commercially used that also *stimulated* the beta-adrenergic receptors as well as

blocked them. Hence, it slows the heart rate less than the other beta-adrenergic blockers, which may be helpful in patients who experience bradycardia (slow heartbeat) with other beta blockers. The drug is used by some doctors to treat heart attacks, tremors, situational anxiety, and antipsychotic(drug)-induced restlessness, in addition to high blood pressure.

Notify your doctor if you have been taking a monoamine oxidase (MAO) inhibitor drug in the past 14 days; if you suffer from diabetes mellitus, asthma, allergic rhinitis (hay fever), emphysema, or congestive heart failure; or your heart beat is below 50 beats per minute. Patients taking insulin, who have fluctuations in the blood sugar, must be closely watched since they may develop dangerously low sugar levels without their usual warning symptoms of rapid heartbeat and sweating. Your blood pressure will probably be closely monitored for the first four weeks to determine if the drug is effective.

You should not take any OTC medication, such as nasal decongestants or cold preparations, unless you check with your doctor or pharmacist first since many of these drugs can cause a rise in your blood pressure. Never increase the dosage of your medication without a doctor's approval. If you miss a dose, take it as soon as possible. However, if the next scheduled dose is within four hours, do not take the missed dose. At no time should you double up on a dose. When preparing to discontinue its use, do not stop abruptly, as that may aggravate the angina or increase risk of a heart attack; reduce its dosage over a one- to two-week period. Use precaution while driving or using machinery that requires alertness or good coordination.

This drug can be taken with meals, if that's convenient. While taking this drug, exercise or heavy exertion may cause lightheadedness. If your heart is prevented from increasing its rate commensurate with your level of activity, your doctor should be consulted to recommend for you an exercise target heart rate. If you are to take a stress test, consult your doctor whether to taper or reduce the level of your medication. Smoking, which is strongly discouraged, can be especially harmful because it can increase the constriction of the lung's bronchial tubes and induce wheezing.

If you take a beta blocker, you should ask your doctor to teach you how to take your pulse. You then can monitor your heart rate before taking a medicine which can lower your rate and cause symptoms of fatigue or dizziness. Additionally, if you have palpitations, you can document the heart rate and rhythm, which helps your doctor make the right diagnosis. It's important that you notify your doctor immediately if you become pregnant when taking a beta-blocker.

Pregnancy

Category B (see page 103). Since this drug appears in breast milk, it is recommended to not nurse while taking it.

Brand Name	Generic Name
LEVATOL	penbutolol
CARTROL	carteolol hydrochloride
	(kar-TEE-o-lol
	hy-dro-KLO-ride)
KERLONE	betaxolol

How These Drugs Work

Reduces blood pressure levels by blocking actions of the sympathetic nervous system; these drugs slow the heart rate, reduce tension in the walls of the blood vessels, and restrict the release by the kidneys of an enzyme called renin.

Purpose

Treatment of hypertension (high blood pressure).

Dosage

Adults: Levatol—20 mg taken orally once daily; maximum dose is 80 mg.

Adults: Cartrol—2.5 mg to 5 mg taken orally once daily; maximum dose is 10 mg.

Adults: Kerlone—10 mg taken orally once daily; maximum dose is 40 mg.

Comments

Levatol (penbutolol), Cartrol (carteolol hydrochloride), and Kerlone (betaxolol) are three relatively new drugs (Kerlone is the most recent) used in the treatment of mild or moderate hypertension and are usually given with other antihypertensive drugs, such as thiazide diuretics. While the action of Levatol and Cartrol are similar to that of other nonselective beta blockers, their side effects are thought to be more mild and less common. Moreover, because these two drugs (along with pindolol and acebutolol) appear to lower blood pressure with less decrease in the heart rate, they are preferred by patients who suffer from symptoms of a slow heartbeat (bradycardia) with other beta blockers. Kerlone (like Lopressor and Tenormin) is cardioselective at lower doses (B1-selective beta blockers) and thus produces less bronchospasm or wheezing in susceptible patients.

Notify your doctor if you have been taking a monoamine oxidase (MAO) inhibitor drug in the past 14 days; suffer from diabetes mellitus, asthma, allergic rhinitis (hay fever), or congestive heart failure; or your heart beat is below 50 beats per minute. Patients taking insulin, who have fluctuations in the blood sugar, must be closely watched since they may develop dangerously low sugar levels without their usual warning symptoms of rapid heartbeat and sweating. Your blood pressure will probably be closely monitored for the first four weeks to determine if the drug is effective.

You should avoid aspirin, or aspirin-containing products, since it could interfere with the drug's effectiveness. Also do not take any OTC medication, such as nasal decongestants or cold preparations, unless you check with your doctor or pharmacist first since many of these drugs can cause a rise in your blood pressure. Never increase the dosage of your medication without a doctor's approval. If you miss a dose, take it as soon as possible. However, if the next scheduled dose is within four hours, do not take the missed dose. At no time should you double up on a dose. It is very important to understand that when preparing to discontinue its use, *do not stop abruptly*, as that may aggravate the angina or increase risk of a heart attack; reduce its dosage over a one- to two-week period. Use precaution while driving or using machinery that requires alertness or good coordination.

While taking this drug, exercise or heavy exertion may cause lightheadedness. If your heart is prevented from increasing its rate commensurate with your level of activity, your doctor should be consulted to recommend for you an exercise target heart rate. If you are to take a stress test, consult your doctor whether to taper or reduce the level of your medication. Smoking, which is strongly discouraged, can be especially harmful because it can increase the constriction of the lung's bronchial tubes and induce wheezing.

If you take a beta blocker, you should ask your doctor to teach you how to take your pulse. You then can monitor your heart rate before taking a medicine which can lower your rate too much and cause symptoms of fatigue or dizziness. Additionally, if you have palpitations (sensation of your heart throbbing) you can document the heart rate and rhythm, which helps your doctor make the right diagnosis. It is important that you notify your doctor immediately if you become pregnant when taking a beta blocker.

Pregnancy
Category C (see page 103).

ALPHA- AND BETA-ADRENERGIC BLOCKERS

Brand Name	*Generic Name*
NORMODYNE,	labetalol hydrochloride
TRANDATE	(la-BET-a-lol
	hy-dro-KLO-ride)

How the Drug Works
Reduces blood pressure levels by blocking actions of the sympathetic nervous system. It slows the heart rate, reduces tension in the walls of the blood vessels, and restricts the release by the kidneys of an enzyme called renin.

Purpose
Treatment of hypertension.

Dosage
Adults: Initially 100 mg taken orally daily in divided doses, followed by an increase of 100 mg after two or three days, if needed. Usual dosage is 200 mg to 400 mg. Patients with severe hypertension may receive increases of 200 mg daily in divided doses up to levels of 600 mg to 1,000 mg. (In hypertensive emergencies, hospitalized patients may receive the drug intravenously.)

Side Effects
Common: Dizziness, fatigue, trouble sleeping, decreased sexual ability.

Uncommon: Anxiety, constipation, diarrhea, headache, nausea, itching of the skin, numbness or tingling of the scalp, changes in taste, stuffy nose, vivid dreams, dry eyes.

Adverse Reactions
Constant fatigue, slow heartbeat, wheezing, depression, hypotension, skin rash, hallucinations, sexual dysfunction, confusion (in elderly).

Drug Interaction
Increases the effects of diuretics.
Cimetidine may increase the effectiveness of labetalol.

Overdosage
If any of the following symptoms develop, a physician should be notified immediately: Slow heartbeat, severe dizziness or fainting, difficulty breathing, seizures.

Comments

Normodyne and Trandate (labetalol) are relatively new drugs used in the treatment of hypertension and combine the benefits of beta blockers and vasodilator drugs. Labetalol hydrochloride is thought to decrease blood pressure more promptly than other beta blockers.

Notify your doctor if you have been taking a monoamine oxidase (MAO) inhibitor drug in the past 14 days; if you suffer from diabetes, chronic bronchitis, asthma, emphysema, or congestive heart failure; or your heartbeat is below 50 beats per minute. Your blood pressure will probably be closely monitored for the first four weeks to determine if the drug is effective.

Although you may experience a stuffy nose while taking this drug, you should not take any OTC medication, such as nasal decongestants or cold preparations, unless you check with your doctor or pharmacist first, since many of these drugs can cause a rise in your blood pressure. Never increase the dosage of your medication without a doctor's approval. If you miss a dose, take it as soon as possible. However, if the next scheduled dose is within four hours, do not take the missed dose. At no time should you take a double dose. When preparing to discontinue its use, do not stop abruptly, as this may aggravate the angina or increase risk of a heart attack; reduce its dosage over a one- to two-week period. Use precaution while driving or using machinery that requires alertness or good coordination.

Avoid excessive salt in your diet, and take the drug about an hour before eating. While taking this drug, exercise or heavy exertion can cause light-headedness; smoking, which is never recommended, can be especially harmful because it can increase the constriction of the bronchial tubes and may reduce the effectiveness of the drug.

Pregnancy

Category C (see page 103). Since the drug appears in breast milk, consult your doctor before you begin breast-feeding.

EIGHT

......

Calcium Antagonists

(Calcium Channel Blockers)

Brand Name	*Generic Name*
CALAN, CALAN SR, ISOPTIN, ISOPTIN SR	verapamil hydrochloride
PROCARDIA	nifedipine
CARDIZEM, CARDIZEM SR	diltiazem hydrochloride

Calcium antagonists prevent the passage of calcium into the cells of the heart and blood vessels, thereby reducing the force of the heart's contractions, relaxing blood vessel pressure, and lowering blood pressure.

Because they increase blood flow while reducing the work load of the heart, these drugs are effective in the treatment of angina—the heart pain that occurs during exercise or is brought on by emotional stress—sometimes alone or in combination with a beta blocker or nitrate. Calcium blockers, beta blockers, and nitrates all play this dual role in the treatment of both hypertension and angina. Calcium blockers are also used to treat heart flutter (atrial arrhythmia) and premature heartbeats.

Among noncardiac problems treatable with calcium blockers are migraine headaches, asthma, and swallowing problems;

Procardia has been used to treat pregnant women beginning early labor.

Potential risks: Calcium blockers can excessively slow the beat of your heart to levels at which you may become very dizzy. Hence, if your pulse rate is below 50 beats per minute, your doctor should not prescribe this type of drug. Moreover, you should not drink alcohol with the drug, never increase its dosage without a doctor's approval, and wait one week between increases. Driving while taking the drug can be risky.

Some patients may experience a swelling of their hands or feet, or a shortness of breath, both of which may indicate cardiac heart failure. By and large these drugs have few other side effects, other than the reported slowed heartbeat. Of the three calcium blockers, verapamil may cause the most heartbeat slowing, while diltiazem may have the lowest risk for this or any other reaction.

Brand Name	*Generic Name*
CALAN, CALAN SR, ISOPTIN, ISOPTIN SR	verapamil (ver-AP-a-mil)

How the Drug Works

By blocking the movement of calcium into the cells of the heart and blood vessels, this drug reduces the force of the heart's contractions and relaxes blood vessels, thereby increasing blood flow while reducing the work load of the heart. By reducing the force of heart muscle contraction, there is less demand for oxygen, thereby reducing angina. Verapamil also slows the heart rate and is effective for arrhythmia.

Purpose

Treatment of angina, both effort-induced and at rest; atrial dysrhythmia (heart flutter); essential hypertension.

Dosage

• Essential hypertension

Adults: Initially 240 mg taken orally in divided doses, with weekly increases up to a maximum of 480 mg daily in divided doses.

• Angina

Adults: Initially 80 mg to 120 mg taken orally three times daily, followed by increases at intervals of seven days if needed up to a maximum dosage of 480 mg daily.

• Atrial dysrhythmia

Adults: 240 mg to 320 mg taken orally in divided doses, three or four times daily.

Side Effects

Common: Dizziness or light-headedness, slow heart rate.

Uncommon: Constipation, dry mouth, flushed skin, headaches, nausea, sweating, blurred vision, impaired urination, fatigue, orthostatic hypotension.

Adverse Reactions

Slow heartbeat, congestive heart failure, edema.

Drug Interaction

Increases the effects of other antihypertensive drugs, digitalis preparations, carbamazepine.

With propranolol and other beta blockers, it may cause heart failure.

Overdosage

If any of the following symptoms develop, notify your physician immediately: Rapid heartbeat, flushed or warm skin, severe dizziness or fainting.

Comments

Introduced in 1967, Calan (verapamil) is used primarily in the treatment of hypertension as a first- or second-line drug in combination with a diuretic or beta blocker. It is also used commonly in the management of angina, alone or in combination with a beta blocker and/or nitrates. The drug can control atrial fibrillation or premature heartbeats and it's also used effectively in the prevention of migraine headaches.

Notify your doctor if you have taken a monoamine oxidase (MAO) inhibitor during the past 14 days, are recovering from a heart attack, have glaucoma, or your pulse rate is below 50 beats per minute. Your blood pressure will probably be closely monitored for the first four weeks to determine if the drug is effective.

You should not take any OTC medication unless you check with your doctor or pharmacist first, since many of these drugs can cause a rise in your blood pressure. Never increase the dosage of your medication without a doctor's approval and make no more than one increase per week. Use precaution while driving or using machinery that requires alertness or good coordination.

Avoid all alcohol and excessive salt in your diet, and take the drug about an hour before eating. If you experience a fever, swelling of your hands or feet, or a shortness of breath, notify your doctor, since these may be signs of cardiac heart failure.

Pregnancy
Category C (see page 103).

Brand Name	*Generic Name*
PROCARDIA	nifedipine
	(ny-FED-i-peen)

How the Drug Works
By blocking the movement of calcium into the cells of the heart and blood vessels, this drug reduces heart contractions and relaxes blood vessels, thereby increasing blood flow while reducing the work load of the heart.

Purpose
Treatment of angina, both effort-induced and at rest.

Dosage
Adults: Initially 10 mg taken orally three times daily, followed by increases as needed. The usual effective dose is 10 mg to 20 mg three times a day; some patients may require 20 mg to 30 mg three times daily. The maximum dosage is 180 mg daily.

Side Effects
Common: Dizziness or light-headedness, flushed skin, headaches, fatigue, nausea, edema.

Uncommon: Constipation, diarrhea, cramps, disturbed sleep, blurred vision, shortness of breath, stuffy nose, sweating, muscle cramps.

Adverse Reactions
Slow heartbeat, fever, congestive heart failure, allergic hepatitis, pulmonary edema.

Drug Interaction
Increases the effects of other antihypertensive drugs and blood thinners.

With propranolol and other beta blockers, it may cause heart failure.

Overdosage
If any of the following symptoms develop, notify your physician immediately: Rapid heartbeat, flushed or warm skin, severe dizziness or fainting.

Comments
Introduced in 1972, Procardia (nifedipine) is used to treat hypertension and the pain of angina. It has many uses, however, including the treatment of high blood pressure, asthma, swallow-

ing problems. In some cases, it is used to treat pregnant women who have gone into early labor.

Notify your doctor if you have taken a monoamine oxidase (MAO) inhibitor during the previous 14 days, are recovering from a heart attack, have glaucoma, or your pulse is below 50 beats per minute. Your blood pressure will probably be closely monitored for the first four weeks to determine if the drug is effective.

You should not take any OTC medication unless you check with your doctor or pharmacist first, since many of these drugs can cause a rise in your blood pressure. Never increase the dosage of your medication without a doctor's approval. If your doctor increases your dosage, the drug may cause temporary anginal pain (which can happen when you first start the drug, as well). If the drug's use is being terminated, its dosage should be reduced slowly to avoid any possible recurrence of the angina. Always swallow the capsule; never crush or chew it. Avoid all alcohol and excessive salt in your diet, and take the drug about an hour before eating.

Pregnancy
Category C (see page 103).

Brand Name	Generic Name
Brand Name CARDIZEM, CARDIZEM SR	*Generic Name* diltiazem hydrochloride (dil-TY-a-zeem)

How the Drug Works
By blocking the movement of calcium into the cells of the heart and blood vessels, this drug reduces heart contractions and relaxes blood vessels, thereby increasing blood flow while reducing the work load of the heart.

Purpose
Treatment of angina.

Dosage
Adults: Cardizem—Initially 30 mg taken orally three to four times daily, before meals and at bedtime, followed if needed by gradual increase every two days to a maximum of 360 mg.

Adults: Cardizem SR (slow release)—Initially 90 mg taken orally twice daily, before a meal and at bedtime, followed if needed by titrating to dosage required; maximum dosage is 360 mg.

Side Effects
Common: Drowsiness, fatigue, edema.

Uncommon: Headaches, nausea, nervousness, insomnia, abdominal cramps, skin rash or flushing, constipation, fatigue, frequent urination, weight gain.

Adverse Reactions
Slow heartbeat, hypotension, arrhythmia, heart block, vomiting, diarrhea, depression, tremor.

Drug Interaction
Increases the effects of digoxin, as well as propranolol and other beta blockers.

Overdosage
If any of the following symptoms develop, notify your physician immediately: Bradycardia (slow heartbeat), hypotension, heart failure.

Comments
Introduced in 1982, Cardizem (diltiazem) is used to treat angina, both effort-associated and at rest, and hypertension. Of all the available calcium blockers, this drug may have the lowest risk of adverse reactions.

Notify your doctor if you have taken a monoamine oxidase (MAO) inhibitor during the past 14 days, are recovering from a heart attack, have glaucoma, or if your pulse is below 50 beats per minute. Your blood pressure will probably be closely monitored for the first four weeks to determine if the drug is effective.

You should not take any OTC medication unless you check with your doctor or pharmacist first, since many of these drugs can cause a rise in your blood pressure. Never increase the dosage of your medication without a doctor's approval and no more than one increase a week. Also, if the drug's use is being terminated dosage should be reduced slowly to avoid any possible recurrence of the angina. Avoid all alcohol and excessive salt in your diet, and take the drug about an hour before eating.

Pregnancy

Category C (see page 103). Since the diltiazem appears in breast milk, consult your doctor before you begin breast-feeding.

NINE
....
Vasodilators

PERIPHERAL VASODILATORS

Brand Name	*Generic Name*
APRESOLINE,	hydralazine
HYDRALAZINE HCI	hydrochloride

ALPHA-1-ADRENERGIC BLOCKERS

Brand Name	*Generic Name*
MINIPRESS	prazosin hydrochloride
HYTRIN	terazosin hydrochloride

ANGIOTENSIN-CONVERTING ENZYME (ACE) INHIBITORS

Brand Name	*Generic Name*
CAPOTEN	captopril
VASOTEC	enalapril maleate

NITRATES

Brand Name	*Generic Name*
NIPRIDE, NITROPRESS	sodium nitroprusside
LONITEN	minoxidil

CENTRAL ALPHA-ADRENERGIC AGONISTS

Brand Name	*Generic Name*
ALDOMET	methyldopa
CATAPRES	clonidine
WYTENSIN	guanabenz acetate
TENEX	guanfacine hydrochloride

PERIPHERAL ADRENERGIC BLOCKERS

Brand Name	*Generic Name*
SERPASIL, SERPALAN	reserpine
HYLOREL	guanadrel sulfate
ISMELIN	guanethidine monosulfate

Vasodilators are drugs that act directly to dilate (widen) the blood vessels, which results in increased blood flow. This is important because high blood pressure—and angina, too, among other ailments—is often the result of narrowing blood vessels. The drugs included in this category are nitrates, angiotensin-converting enzyme (ACE) inhibitors, and sympatholytics. However, since by definition vasodilators are drugs that improve blood flow by dilating blood vessels, calcium channel blockers could also be considered vasodilators.

Because the size of your blood vessels is influenced by a variety of mechanisms, vasodilators act on the different ways to control the width of the vessel: alpha-1 adrenergic blockers (Apresoline and Minipress) inhibit the contraction of the muscles in the lining of the blood vessels by interfering with nerve signals to the muscles; ACE inhibitors (Capoten and Vasotec) block the activity of a naturally occurring enzyme in your blood, angiotensin, allowing the vessel to dilate; and nitrates (Nipride) act directly on the muscles of the lining to produce the same results.

Potential risks: The primary risk is that some of these powerful vasodilators may be too effective, and your blood pressure might fall too low. Hence, your doctor will carefully monitor your use of these powerful drugs. Most other problems related to their use are far less serious, such as the possibility of edema, light-headedness, and headaches. When used as directed by your doctor, however, vasodilators play an important role in the treatment of high blood pressure, especially severe hypertension.

PERIPHERAL VASODILATORS

Brand Name	*Generic Name*
APRESOLINE,	hydralazine
HYDRALAZINE HCI	hydrochloride
	(hy-DRAL-a-zeen
	hy-dro-KLO-ride)

How the Drug Works

By relaxing the blood vessels, it widens (dilates) the blood vessels, thereby lowering blood pressure and increasing the flow of blood.

Purpose

Treatment of hypertension and heart failure.

Dosage

Adults: Initially 10 mg taken orally given four times daily for first two to four days, followed by increases up to 25 mg for first week, followed by increases up to 50 mg four times daily. Recommended maximum dosage is 200 mg, but some patients may require dosages of 300 mg or 400 mg daily. (Dosage will have to be modified for patients with kidney disease.)

Children: Initially 0.75 mg taken orally in four divided doses, followed by gradual increases over a month to a maximum of 200 mg daily.

Side Effects

Common: Diarrhea, headache, nausea and vomiting, anorexia, heart palpitations.

Uncommon: Stuffy nose, constipation, tearing eyes or conjunctivitis, flushing, dizziness.

Adverse Reactions

Chest pain, skin rash, difficult urination, edema, chills, joint pain, persistent fatigue.

Rare: Hepatitis.

Drug Interaction

Increases the effects of other antihypertensives, including diuretics and monoamine oxidase (MAO) inhibitors.

With diazoxide (administered only intravenously), it can cause severe hypotension (low blood pressure).

Overdosage

If any of the following symptoms develop, a physician should be notified immediately: Severe hypotension, rapid heartbeat, headache, cold and sweaty skin, extreme weakness, arrhythmia, shock.

Comments

Apresoline (hydralazine hydrochloride), often referred to as a vasodilator, has been around since 1952. It is usually given after other treatments have been unable to lower blood pressure and generally in conjunction with other drugs, such as a diuretic to reduce the side effect of fluid retention and a beta blocker to prevent rapid heartbeat. When this drug is given alone it decreases diastolic pressure more than systolic pressure (see page 28).

Notify your doctor if you have been taking a monoamine oxidase (MAO) inhibitor (an antihypertensive drug) within the past two weeks, are recovering from a heart attack, have glaucoma or a history of liver or kidney disease, or if your pulse is below 50 beats per minute. Your blood pressure will probably be closely monitored for the first four weeks to determine if the drug is effective and your eyes may be examined periodically as well.

Initially, you may feel drowsy or run down with this drug, but those effects should wear off as soon your body grows accustomed to the lowered blood pressure during the few first weeks. If you move slowly while changing positions, especially if rising from a sitting or lying position, it will reduce the likelihood of dizziness. You may experience headaches if you have a history of migraines. The drug is designed to make each contraction of your heart more forceful, so you may experience a pounding heartbeat. As your blood pressure is reduced, your heart rate may increase. As with all antihypertensive medications, it is advised that you keep a record of your pulse so that if any symptoms develop you have a pulse history to report to your doctor.

Do not stop taking this drug without your doctor's approval and never stop abruptly, since it can cause a sharp rise in your blood pressure. It is advised that you gradually reduce your dosage over a two- to four-day period. If you miss a scheduled dose, do not double your next dose. You should not take any OTC medication, such as nasal decongestants or cold preparations, unless you check with your doctor or pharmacist, since many of these drugs can cause a rise in your blood pressure. Never increase the dosage of your medication without a doctor's approval. It is best to take the drug with meals so to increase its absorption. Use precaution while driving or using machinery that requires alertness or good coordination.

Avoid drinking alcohol, as it may exaggerate the effects of the drug. If you begin to retain salt and water with the drug's use, your doctor can prescribe a diuretic (Chapter 6). If you experience fever, sore throat, or muscle or joint pain, call your doctor immediately, as these may be signs that you are having an adverse reaction. A simple blood test can verify if these symptoms are related to your use of the drug. If you are bothered by dry mouth, sugarless gum or hard candy can give you relief.

Pregnancy
Category C (see page 103).

ALPHA-1-ADRENERGIC BLOCKERS

Brand Name
MINIPRESS

Generic Name
prazosin hydrochloride
(PRAZ-o-sin
hy-dro-KLO-ride)

How the Drug Works

By blocking the alpha-1-adrenergic receptors in the brain and spinal cord, which ordinarily are stimulated by adrenaline to constrict the muscles of the blood vessels, it dilates (widens) both blood veins and arteries to increase the flow of blood and lower blood pressure.

Purpose

Treatment of hypertension and heart failure.

Dosage

Adults: Initially 1 mg taken orally each day, followed by increases up to 20 mg in divided doses; the usual maintenance dose is 6 mg to 15 mg daily in divided doses.

Side Effects

Common: Dizziness, drowsiness, dry mouth, fatigue.

Uncommon: Nausea and vomiting, palpitations, blurred vision, sudden fainting.

Among the elderly: Light-headedness, fainting.

Adverse Reactions

Chest pain, weight gain, difficult urination, edema, numbness in hands or feet, depression, shortness of breath, impotence, priapism.

Drug Interaction

Increases the effects of other antihypertensives, especially beta blockers.

Overdosage

If any of the following symptoms develop, notify your physician immediately: Poor reflexes, severe hypotension, cold sweaty skin, persistent drowsiness.

Comments

Minipress (prazozin hydrochloride), introduced in 1975, was very popular among many physicians, but is used less often now because of its side effects. It is usually not given as the first drug, but as a "Step 2" medication, generally in conjunction with other antihypertensive drugs.

Notify your doctor if you have been taking a monoamine oxidase (MAO) inhibitor within the past two weeks, are recovering from a stroke, have a history of depression or heart, liver, or kidney disease. Initially you may feel drowsy or run down with this drug, or you may also experience a sudden fainting sensation during the first week of your drug therapy. The sudden fainting is called "first dose syncope." If you feel faint within the first hour or so after taking the drug, your doctor may recommend that you take a single dose before going to bed at night. Once your body grows accustomed to the lowered blood pressure, however, these side effects should cease. If you move slowly while changing positions, especially if rising from a sitting or lying position, it will reduce the likelihood of any dizziness. If you take your medicine just before going to bed, be especially careful if you need to get up during the night. For the same reasons, use precaution while driving or using machinery that requires alertness or good coordination.

Do not stop taking this drug without your doctor's approval and never stop abruptly, since this can cause a sharp rise in your blood pressure. It is advised that you gradually reduce your dosage over a two- to four-day period. You should not take any OTC medication unless you check with your doctor or pharmacist first, since many of these drugs can cause a rise in your blood pressure. Never increase the dosage of your medication without a doctor's approval. Your blood pressure will probably be closely monitored for the first four weeks to determine if the drug is effective. Avoid drinking alcohol as it may exaggerate the effects of the drug. If you are bothered by dry mouth, sugarless gum or hard candy can give you relief.

Pregnancy

Category C (see page 103). Since the drug appears in breast milk, consult your doctor before you begin breast-feeding.

Brand Name
HYTRIN

Generic Name
terazosin hydrochloride
(te-RAZ-o-sin
hy-dro-KLO-ride)

How the Drug Works

By blocking the alpha and adrenergic receptors, it dilates (widens) blood veins and arteries to increase the flow of blood and lower blood pressure.

Purpose

Treatment of hypertension.

Dosage

Adults: Initially 1 mg taken orally at bedtime, followed by gradual increases up to 20 mg in a single dose; the usual maintenance dose is 1 mg to 5 mg per day.

Side Effects

Common: Dizziness, headaches, weakness and fatigue, stuffy nose.

Uncommon: Palpitations, weight gain, constipation.

Adverse Reactions

Chest pain, back pain, difficult urination, swelling (edema) or pain in the hands and legs, nausea and vomiting, blurred vision, dyspnea, depression.

Drug Interaction

Increases the effects of other antihypertensives.

Overdosage

If any of the following symptoms develop, notify your physician immediately: Tachycardia (rapid heartbeat), severe hypotension.

Comments

Hytrin (terazosin hydrochloride), like Minipress, is a centrally acting vasodilator and is usually given as a "Step 2" medication, generally in conjunction with other antihypertensive drugs.

Notify your doctor if you have been taking a monoamine oxidase (MAO) inhibitor within the past two weeks, are recovering from a stroke, or have a history of depression or heart, liver, or kidney disease.

Initially, you may feel drowsy or run down with this drug, and you may also experience a sudden fainting sensation during the first week of your drug therapy ("first dose syncope"). For this reason the drug should first be given at bedtime and the initial dose should not exceed 1 mg. Once your body grows accustomed to the lowered blood pressure, however, these side effects should cease. Do not stop taking the drug without your doctor's approval and never stop abruptly since it can cause a sharp rise in your blood pressure. It is advised that you gradually reduce your dosage over a two- to four-day period. If you discontinue the use of this drug for several days, again under your doctor's supervision, you will need to return to a 1 mg dose and be retitrated (see "Titration," page 68).

If you move slowly while changing positions, especially if rising from a sitting or lying position, it will reduce the likelihood of any dizziness. If you take your medicine just before going to bed, be especially careful if you need to get up during the night. For the same reasons, use precaution while driving or using machinery that requires alertness or good coordination.

You should not take any OTC medication unless you check with your doctor or pharmacist first, since many of these drugs can cause a rise in your blood pressure. Never increase the dosage of your medication without a doctor's approval. Your blood pressure will probably be closely monitored for the first four weeks to determine if the drug is effective. Avoid drinking alcohol, as it may exaggerate the effects of the drug. If you are bothered by dry mouth, sugarless gum or hard candy can give you relief.

Pregnancy
Category C (see page 103). Since the drug appears in breast milk, consult your doctor before you begin breast-feeding.

ANGIOTENSIN-CONVERTING ENZYME (ACE) INHIBITORS

Brand Name	*Generic Name*
CAPOTEN	captopril (CAP-to-pril)

How the Drug Works
Lowers blood pressure by inhibiting the release of angiotensin, an enzyme that constricts the blood vessels and probably causes sodium and fluid retention.

Purpose
Treatment of hypertension and congestive heart failure.

Dosage
• Hypertension
Adults: Initially 6.25 mg taken orally two or three times daily, and increased gradually, if necessary, to 50 mg three times daily. If blood pressure must be further reduced, dosage may reach 100 mg to 150 mg, usually with a diuretic. Maximum dosage is 450 mg daily.
• Congestive heart failure
Adults: Initially 6.25 mg taken orally three times daily, increased to 25 mg three times daily in conjunction with other

congestive heart failure drugs. Dosage levels may reach 100 mg to 150 mg if necessary.

Side Effects
Common: Loss of taste, persistent cough, dizziness, constipation.

Adverse Reactions
Palpitations, difficult breathing, fever, sore throat, swelling of hands or feet, rash, itchy skin, frequent urination, chest pains, angina, fever, faintness, significant reduction in white blood cells (creating susceptibility to fever and infection).

Drug Interaction
Increases the effects of other antihypertensive medications.

In combination with a potassium-retaining drug (e.g., Dyazide), it may cause a dangerous accumulation of potassium in the blood.

Overdosage
If any of the following symptoms develop, notify your physician immediately: Severe dizziness or faintness.

Comments
Capoten (captopril) is a potent antihypertensive drug that works quickly. Capoten causes fewer side effects and produces a better "quality of life" profile than beta blockers and diuretics. In addition to hypertension, this drug is also used on occasions to treat rheumatoid arthritis and certain types of kidney disease and edema. Studies have also shown that ACE inhibitors such as Capoten and Vasotec may not be as effective in black patients as in white.

Your doctor may give you a test dose of 6.25 mg to exclude the possibility that another medical condition is the cause of your hypertension (e.g., kidney disease). If your blood pressure cannot be reduced successfully with this drug alone, your doctor may add a modest dose of a thiazide diuretic (see Chapter 6) and increase its dose until your blood pressure is reduced successfully. Only if this combination is unsuccessful will your doctor increase the Capoten to levels of 100 mg or more.

This drug should be used cautiously if you suffer a serious autoimmune disease or have a history of heart disease, stroke, or liver or kidney disease.

You may experience a sudden fainting sensation during the first week of your drug therapy. If you move slowly while changing positions, especially if rising from a sitting or lying position, it will reduce the likelihood of any dizziness. Also, excessive perspiration or dehydration can lead to a fall in blood pressure. You may also feel drowsy or run down with this drug for the first week or two. One of the most disturbing side effects of Capoten is a persistent dry, nonproductive cough, which may necessitate a reduction in the dosage level or possibly discontinuation of the drug.

Never increase the dosage of your medication without a doctor's approval. If you miss a dose, take it as soon as possible, and then resume your regular schedule. Do not stop taking this drug without your doctor's approval and never stop abruptly, since this can cause a sharp rise on your blood pressure. Your blood pressure will probably be closely monitored for the first four weeks to determine if the drug is effective. Notify your doctor if you develop a fever, sore throat, mouth sores, or any sign of an infection. Women must also notify their doctor if they become pregnant while using this drug.

Do not take any OTC medication unless you check with your doctor or pharmacist first, since many of these drugs can cause a rise in your blood pressure. Do not take the drug immediately before or following a meal, for a full stomach can interfere with the drug's absorption. Rather, it is advised to take the drug at least one hour before or two hours following a meal.

Pregnancy

Category C (see page 103). Since the drug appears in breast milk, consult your doctor before you begin breast-feeding.

Brand Name	*Generic Name*
VASOTEC*	enalapril maleate
	(e-NAL-a-pril
	MAL-ee-ate)

How the Drug Works

Lowers blood pressure by inhibiting the release of angiotensin, an enzyme that constricts the blood vessels and probably causes sodium and fluid retention.

Purpose

Treatment of hypertension and congestive heart failure.

Dosage

Adults: Initially 5 mg taken orally daily; and if necessary, dosage can be increased to 10 mg to 40 mg daily in a single or divided dose.

Side Effects

Common: Loss of taste, persistent cough, headache, dizziness, fatigue.

Uncommon: Insomnia, nervousness, diarrhea, nausea.

Adverse Reactions

Difficult breathing; fever; sore throat; swelling of the face, eyes, lips, tongue (angioedema); rash; itchy skin; frequent urination; palpitations; faintness.

Rare: Chest pains.

---

* The following drugs, with their generic names in parentheses, are angiotensin converting enzyme (ACE) inhibitors that have recently been approved for hypertension, though your doctor may also prescribe them for congestive heart failure: Lotensin (benazapril), Monopril (fosinopril), Prinivil, Zestril (lisinopril), Accupril (quinapril), Altace (ramipril). While their dosages may vary, these newer drugs may offer no significant advantages over currently available ACE inhibitors. Their side effect profile and drug interactions are similar to Capoten (see page 189) and Vasotec.

Drug Interaction
With lithium, may cause lithium toxicity.

Overdosage
If any of the following symptoms develop, notify your physician immediately: Severe dizziness or faintness.

Comments
Vasotec (enalapril maleate) is an antihypertensive drug that has a reputation of providing more sustained action than Capoten, so some people may only have to take it once a day. In addition to hypertension, it is also used on occasions to treat childhood hypertension. Studies have also shown that ACE inhibitors such as Vasotec and Capoten may not be as effective in black patients as in white.

If you are taking any other hypertensive drug, and especially a diuretic, your doctor will have you stop taking that drug for two or three days before you start this drug. If your blood pressure is not reduced with this drug alone, your doctor may then prescribe a diuretic. This drug should be used cautiously if you suffer from diabetes or have a history of heart disease, stroke, or liver or kidney disease.

One of the most disturbing side effects of Vasotec is a persistent dry, nonproductive cough, which may necessitate a reduction in the dosage level or possibly discontinuation of the drug. You may also feel drowsy or run down with this drug. You may also experience a sudden fainting sensation during the first week of your drug therapy. If you move slowly while changing position, especially if rising from a sitting or lying position, it will reduce the likelihood of any dizziness.

Never increase the dosage of your medication without a doctor's approval. If you miss a dose, take it as soon as possible, and then resume your regular schedule. Do not stop taking this drug without your doctor's approval and never stop abruptly, since it can cause a sharp rise in your blood pressure.

Your blood pressure, along with occasional blood samples, may be monitored for the first four weeks to determine if the drug is effective. Notify your doctor if you develop a fever, sore throat, or any sign of an infection. Women must also notify their doctor if they become pregnant while using this drug.

Do not take any OTC medication unless you check with your doctor or pharmacist first, since many of these drugs can cause a rise in your blood pressure. A full stomach can interfere with the drug's absorption, so do not take the drug immediately before or following a meal. Rather, it is advised to take the drug at least one hour before or two hours following a meal.

Pregnancy
Category C (see page 103).

NITRATES

Brand Name	*Generic Name*
NIPRIDE, NITROPRESS	sodium nitroprusside
	(NY-tro-prus-ide)

How the Drug Works
By dilating (widening) the blood veins and arteries, it increases the flow of blood and lowers blood pressure.

Purpose
Treatment of hypertension, especially in a hypertensive crisis.

Dosage
Adults and children: 3 mcg/kg/minute, administered intravenously.

Side Effects
Common: Hypotension, rapid heartbeat.
Uncommon: If administered too rapidly, excessively reduced blood pressure, nausea, headache, palpitations, chest pains.

Adverse Reactions

With prolonged usage, ringing in the ears, confusion, blurred vision, anemia, convulsions. Nipride is metabolized to cyanide and its metabolite thiocyanate; if levels of thiocyanate are elevated for several days, side effects could include nausea, fatigue, and psychosis. The treatment for cyanide poisoning is administration of sodium thiosulfate or hydroxocobalamin.

Drug Interaction

Because it is a potent vasodilator, Nipride *increases* the effects of other antihypertensive agents.

Overdosage

If any of the following symptoms develop, a physician should be notified immediately: Profound hypotension and cyanide poisoning.

Comments

Because of its potency, Nipride is administered only intravenously under close medical supervision, and usually only during a hypertensive emergency, when blood pressure must be brought under control immediately.

Pregnancy

Category C (see page 103).

Brand Name	*Generic Name*
LONITEN	minoxidil (mi-NOX-i-dil)

How the Drug Works

By dilating (widening) the blood veins and arteries, it increases the flow of blood and lowers blood pressure.

Purpose

Treatment of severe hypertension.

Dosage

Adults: Initially 5 mg taken orally daily as a single dose, followed by increases to 10 mg, 20 mg, and then 40 mg in single or divided doses; maximum dosage is 100 mg.

Children under 12 years of age: 0.2 mg daily in single dose, followed by increases in increments of 0.25 mg to 1 mg. Maximum dosage is 50 mg. Some suggest a 100 mg maximum dosage.

Side Effects

Common: Increased hair growth on face, arms, and back; orthostatic hypotension (dizziness when rising from a sitting or lying position).

Uncommon: Breast tenderness in males and females, headaches.

Adverse Reactions

Common: Rapid heartbeat, weight gain, chest pain, shortness of breath.

Uncommon: Bloating, flushed skin, swelling of the lower legs.

Rare: Skin rash; itching; numbness or tingling of face, hands, or feet.

Drug Interaction

Increases the hypotensive effect of guanethidine.

Overdosage

If any of the following symptoms develop, notify your physician immediately: Severe hypotension, rapid heartbeat, extreme weakness.

Comments

Loniten (minoxidil), introduced in 1972, is a potent, long-acting antihypertensive that is usually given only after other treatments have been unable to lower blood pressure and usually in combination with a diuretic to reduce the side effect of fluid retention and a beta blocker to prevent rapid heartbeat. In addition to edema or fluid retention, the drug can also increase the pain of angina. Hence, notify your doctor if either of these symptoms develop, especially if you have an existing coronary disease.

Another drawback in minoxidil's use is the frequent and dramatic growth in hair—both longer and darker than is usual—that occurs in well over half of all patients who take this drug for more than one month. After the drug's discontinuation, however, the new hair growth ceases and, over a few weeks or months, gradually disappears. Do not stop taking this drug without your doctor's approval and never stop abruptly, since this can cause a sharp rise in your blood pressure. It is advised that you gradually reduce your dosage over a two- to four-day period. If you miss a scheduled dose, do not double your next dose.

Notify your doctor if you have been taking the antihypertensive drug guanethidine monosulfate (Ismelin), since in combination the two can cause a sharp drop in blood pressure. Moreover, notify your doctor if you have lupus or a history of heart, liver, or kidney disease. Your blood pressure will probably be closely monitored for the first four weeks to determine if the drug is effective. It is also advised that you take your pulse at regular intervals during the day; if your resting pulse (without exercise or exertion) has increased 20 beats or more, notify your doctor. Furthermore, weigh yourself weekly and report any weight gain of more than 5 pounds.

You should not take any OTC medication, such as nasal decongestants or cold preparations, unless you check with your doctor or pharmacist first, since many of these drugs can cause a rise in your blood pressure. Never increase the dosage of your medication without a doctor's approval. Avoid drinking alcohol, as it may exaggerate the effects of the drug.

Pregnancy
Category C (see page 103).

CENTRAL ALPHA-ADRENERGIC AGONISTS

Brand Name	*Generic Name*
ALDOMET	methyldopa
	(meth-il-DO-pa)

How the Drug Works
By inhibiting the activity of the nerves that control the muscles in the walls of the blood vessels, it widens (dilates) the blood vessels, thus lowering blood pressure and increasing the flow of blood.

Purpose
Treatment of hypertension.

Dosage
Adults: Initially 250 mg taken orally in divided doses (two or three times daily) for the first 48 hours, followed by increases every few days in divided doses, or possibly the entire dosage at bedtime, up to a maximum of 3 grams daily. Maintenance dosage is 500 mg to 2 grams daily in divided doses.

Children: Initially 10 mg taken orally in divided doses (two to four times daily), followed by daily increases up to a maximum of 65 mg if needed.

Side Effects
Common: Dry mouth, headaches, drowsiness, lethargy.

Uncommon: Diarrhea, skin rash, stuffy nose, nausea, vomiting, lack of sexual interest or impotence, swelling of the breasts, lactorrhea, flatulence.

Adverse Reactions
Edema in lower legs and feet, depression, fever, anxiety, vivid dreams, orthostatic hypertension (dizziness when rising from a sitting or lying position), weight gain.

Drug Interaction

Increases the effects of other antihypertensive drugs or oral anticoagulants.

Overdosage

If any of the following symptoms develop, notify your physician immediately: Severe dizziness or fainting; confusion; weak pulse; diarrhea, nausea, and vomiting.

Comments

Introduced in 1963, Aldomet (methyldopa) is usually given as a "Step 2" medication, often in conjunction with other antihypertensive drugs including a diuretic. It is used less frequently now that calcium antagonists (see Chapter 8) and ACE inhibitors (see page 189) have also become popular. Women who develop pregnancy-related hypertension are prescribed methyldopa as it is considered quite safe. People who are sensitive or have had allergic reactions to sulfur should ask their doctor or pharmacist whether the particular preparation of Aldomet contains sulfite preservatives.

Lower doses may be necessary in the elderly. Your blood levels may be monitored for the first few weeks of use, and your doctor may order periodic liver function tests during the first three months to ensure safe and effective use.

Initially, you may feel drowsy or run down with methyldopa, but those effects should wear off as soon your body grows accustomed to the lowered blood pressure, after a few weeks. If you move slowly when changing positions, especially if rising from a sitting or lying position, it will reduce the likelihood of dizziness. You should not take any OTC medication, such as nasal decongestants or cold preparations, unless you check with your doctor or pharmacist first, since many of these drugs can cause a rise in your blood pressure. You may feel depressed for periods while taking the drug. The symptoms include early-morning awakening, listlessness, fatigue, and increased irritability.

Never increase the dosage of your medication without a doctor's approval, but if you miss a scheduled dose, take it as soon as possible and then resume your regular schedule. Use precaution while driving or using machinery that requires alertness or good coordination.

Avoid all alcohol and excessive salt in your diet. You may experience some weight gain, at least initially. If you begin to retain salt and water, your doctor can prescribe a diuretic. If you experience a fever or any other adverse reactions, notify your doctor. When preparing to discontinue its use, do not stop abruptly, as this may aggravate the angina or increase risk of a heart attack; reduce its dosage over a one- to two-week period. If you are bothered by dry mouth, try sugarless gum or hard candy for relief.

Pregnancy

Category B (see page 103). Since the drug appears in breast milk, it is advised that you stop breast-feeding while taking this drug.

Brand Name	*Generic Name*
CATAPRES	clonidine (KLON-i-deen)

How the Drug Works

By inhibiting the activity of the nerves that control the muscles in the walls of the blood vessels, it widens (dilates) the blood vessels, thus lowering blood pressure and increasing the flow of blood.

Purpose

Treatment of hypertension and high blood pressure.

Dosage

Adults: Initially 0.1 mg taken orally, followed by increments of 0.1 or 0.2 mg daily up to a maximum of 2.4 mg daily; maintenance dosage is usually 0.2 mg to 0.8 mg daily, given in divided doses.

Side Effects
Common: Dry mouth, dizziness, drowsiness.

Uncommon: Orthostatic hypotension (dizziness when rising from a sitting or lying position); constipation; dry or irritated eyes; nausea; vomiting; urinary retention; lack of sexual interest, or impotence; weight gain.

Adverse Reactions
Depression; nightmares; anxiety; chest pains; headache; cold fingers and feet, or a tingling, burning sensation in the extremities; restlessness; stomach cramps; irregular heartbeats.

Drug Interaction
Increases the effects of other antihypertensive drugs or central nervous system (CNS) depressants, including sedatives and alcohol, and antihistamines.

Tricyclic antidepressants and MAO inhibitors may decrease effectiveness of this drug.

With Propranolol and other beta blockers, it can cause increased hypertension.

Overdosage
If any of the following symptoms develop, notify your physician immediately: Severe dizziness or fainting, weakness, difficult breathing, slow heartbeat, vomiting.

Comments
Catapres (clonidine) was introduced in Europe in 1963 and in this country in 1974. It is used most often as a "Step 2" medication, often in conjunction with another antihypertensive drug. It has been used successfully in the prevention of migraine headaches and for the treatment of dysmenorrhea, which is painful or difficult menstruation, as well as high blood pressure. This drug is also available in transdermal patches (Catapres-TTS) that can be applied once weekly.

It is very important not to stop taking this drug without your doctor's approval and never to stop abruptly, since this can cause a sharp rise in your blood pressure. Abrupt withdrawal may trigger a *rebound hypertension* that occurs when the nerve receptors are suddenly bombarded by stimulation. Therefore, discuss any change in dosage or adverse reaction carefully with your doctor. In addition, if you are entering a hospital, notify your new doctor not only of this drug but of all your medications so there will be no discontinuation of therapy. When discontinuing this drug, it is advised that you gradually reduce your dosage over a two- to four-day period.

Initially, you may feel drowsy or run down with this drug, but those effects should wear off as soon as your body grows accustomed to the lowered blood pressure, during the few first weeks. If you move slowly when changing position, especially if rising from a sitting or lying position, it will reduce the likelihood of dizziness.

Notify your doctor if you have been taking a monoamine oxidase (MAO) inhibitor (an antihypertensive drug) within the past two weeks, are recovering from a heart attack or have glaucoma, or if your pulse is below 50 beats per minute. Your blood pressure will probably be closely monitored for the first four weeks to determine if the drug is effective and your eyes may be examined periodically as well.

You should not take any OTC medication, such as nasal decongestants or cold preparations, unless you check with your doctor or pharmacist first, since many of these drugs can cause a rise in your blood pressure. Never increase the dosage of your medication without a doctor's approval and make no more than one increase a week. If you miss a scheduled dose, take it as soon as possible and then resume your regular schedule. It is best to take the last dose just before going to bed. Use precaution while driving or using machinery that requires alertness or good coordination.

If you begin to retain salt and water, your doctor can prescribe a diuretic. If you are bothered by dry mouth, try sugarless gum or hard candy for relief.

Pregnancy
Category C (see page 103). Since the drug appears in breast milk, it is advised that you stop breast-feeding while taking this drug.

———

Brand Name	*Generic Name*
WYTENSIN	guanabenz acetate
	(GWAN-a-benz
	ASS-e-tate)

How the Drug Works
By inhibiting the activity of the nerves that control the muscles in the walls of the blood vessels, it widens (dilates) the blood vessels and, thereby, lowers blood pressure and increases the flow of blood.

Purpose
Treatment of hypertension.

Dosage
Adults: Initially 4 mg taken orally twice daily, followed if necessary by increases in increments of 4 mg or 8 mg daily every one to two weeks, up to 32 mg twice daily.

Side Effects
Common: Drowsiness, dizziness, dry mouth, headaches, fatigue.
Uncommon: Decreased sexual ability, nausea, constipation, blurred vision.

Adverse Reactions
Depression, nightmares, insomnia, anxiety, chest pains, palpitations, irregular heart beats, breast enlargement.

Drug Interaction

Increases the effects of other antihypertensive drugs or central nervous system (CNS) depressants, including sedatives and alcohol and antihistamines.

Overdosage

If any of the following symptoms develop, notify your physician immediately: Severe dizziness or fainting, weakness.

Comments

Wytensin (guanabenz) is used both alone and with a diuretic. It is very important that you not stop taking this drug without your doctor's approval and never stop abruptly, since this can cause a sharp rise in your blood pressure. Abrupt withdrawal may trigger a *rebound hypertension*, when the nerve receptors are suddenly bombarded by stimulation. Therefore, discuss any change in dosage or adverse reaction carefully with your doctor. In addition, if you are entering a hospital, notify your new doctor not only of this drug but of all your medications so there will be no discontinuation of therapy. When discontinuing this drug, it is advised that you gradually reduce your dosage over a two- to four-day period.

Initially, you may feel drowsy or run down with this drug, but those effects should wear off as soon as your body grows accustomed to the lowered blood pressure, during the few first weeks. Rising slowly from a sitting or lying position will reduce the likelihood of dizziness. Avoid alcohol while taking this drug, as it may cause excessive drowsiness. If you are bothered by a dry mouth, try chewing sugarless gum or hard candy for relief.

Notify your doctor if you have been taking a monoamine oxidase (MAO) inhibitor (antihypertensive drug) within the past two weeks, are recovering from a heart attack, or have glaucoma, or if your pulse is below 50 beats per minute. Your blood pressure will probably be closely monitored for the first four weeks to determine if the drug is effective, and your eyes may be examined periodically as well.

You should not take any OTC medication, such as nasal decongestants or cold preparations, unless you check with your doctor or pharmacist first, since many of these drugs can cause a rise in your blood pressure. Never increase the dosage of your medication without a doctor's approval, and make no more than one increase a week. If you miss a scheduled dose, take it as soon as possible and then resume your regular schedule. It is best to take the last dose just before going to bed. Use precaution while driving or using machinery that requires alertness or good coordination.

Pregnancy
Category C (see page 103).

Brand Name
TENEX

Generic Name
guanfacine hydrochloride
(GWAN-fa-seen
hy-dro-KLO-ride)

How the Drug Works
By inhibiting the activity of the nerves that control the muscles in the walls of the blood vessels, it widens (dilates) the blood vessels, thus lowering blood pressure and increasing the flow of blood.

Purpose
Treatment of hypertension in those already receiving a thiazide diuretic.

Dosage
Adults: Initially 1 mg taken orally at bedtime; if results are not satisfactory after three to four weeks, doses of 2 mg and then 3 mg a day may be given. Doses may also be divided.

Side Effects
Common: Dizziness, drowsiness, dry mouth, headaches, insomnia, constipation, lethargy.

Uncommon: Diarrhea, skin rash, stuffy nose, nausea, vomiting, lack of sexual interest or impotence (at 3 mg per day).

Adverse Reactions
Bradycardia (rapid heartbeat), palpitations, depression, orthostatic hypertension (dizziness when rising from a sitting or lying position), leg cramps.

Drug Interaction
Increases the effects of central nervous system (CNS) depressants, such as alcohol and barbiturates.

Overdosage
If any of the following symptoms develop, notify your physician immediately: Severe dizziness or fainting; confusion; weak pulse; diarrhea, nausea, and vomiting.

Comments
Tenex (guanfacine hydrochloride) is usually given as a "Step 2" medication, often in conjunction with other antihypertensive drugs including a diuretic. It is considered as effective as the other central alpha-adrenergic drugs, but its effects last longer ("longer duration of action") which permits most patients to take it only once daily, usually at bedtime. Its adverse effects are considered milder than those of clonidine.

Your blood levels may be monitored for the first few weeks of use, and your doctor may order periodic liver function tests during the first three months to ensure safe and effective use. Initially, you may feel drowsy or run down with this drug, but those effects should wear off as soon as your body grows accustomed to the lowered blood pressure, during the few first weeks. Rising slowly from a sitting or lying position will reduce the likelihood of dizziness. You should not take any OTC medication, such as nasal decongestants or cold preparations, unless you check with your doctor or pharmacist first, since many of these drugs can cause a rise in your blood pressure. You may feel depressed for periods while you are taking the drug.

Never increase the dosage of your medication without a doctor's approval, but if you miss a scheduled dose, take it as soon as possible and then resume your regular schedule. Use precaution while driving or using machinery that requires alertness or good coordination.

Avoid all alcohol and excessive salt in your diet. If you begin to retain salt and water with this drug's use, your doctor can prescribe a diuretic. When preparing to discontinue its use, do not stop abruptly, as this may aggravate angina or increase risk of a heart attack; reduce its dosage over a one- to two-week period. If you are bothered by dry mouth, try sugarless gum or hard candy for relief.

Pregnancy

Category B (see page 103). Since the drug appears in breast milk, it is advised that you stop breast-feeding while taking it.

PERIPHERAL ADRENERGIC BLOCKERS

Brand Name
SERPASIL, SERPALAN,
   (and many other brand
   names)

Generic Name
reserpine (re-SER-peen)

How the Drug Works

By inhibiting the release of the neurotransmitter norepinephrine, which controls nerve impulses, it reduces the tension in the walls of the blood vessels and lowers blood pressure.

Purpose

Treatment of mild to moderate hypertension.

Dosage

Adults: 0.1 mg to 0.25 mg (taken orally) daily.
Children: 5 to 20 mcg (taken orally) daily.

Side Effects

Common: Dry mouth, dizziness, diarrhea, loss of appetite, nausea, nasal congestion, slow heartbeat.

Uncommon: Decreased sexual interest or impotence in males.

Adverse Reactions

Faintness, constant fatigue, anxiety, vivid dreams, early morning insomnia, tarry stools, swelling of feet and lower legs, chest pain, breast enlargement, acid indigestion or stomach cramps.

RARE: Painful urination, skin rash, trembling hands or feet, signs of easy bruising, loss of scalp hair, nighttime urination.

Drug Interaction

Increases the effects of other antihypertensives and sedatives. *With MAO inhibitors,* it may cause hypertension.

Overdosage

If any of the following symptoms develop, notify your physician immediately: Severe dizziness or drowsiness, fainting, cold and sweaty skin, flushed skin, severe diarrhea.

Comments

Serpasil (reserpine), which has been around since 1952, is used less frequently than in the past because of its side effects. It is usually used only after a first step treatment with a diuretic or beta blocker alone has not been successful. (However, reserpine may be used in combination with a thiazide diuretic as a "Step 1" medication as well.

Notify your doctor if you have been taking a monoamine oxidase (MAO) inhibitor within the past two weeks, or suffer from depression, a peptic ulcer, or ulcerative colitis. It should also be used cautiously if you have a history of heart disease, seizures, gallstones, or liver or kidney disease.

Initially, you may feel drowsy or run down with this drug, or you may experience a sudden fainting sensation during the first week of your drug therapy. If you move slowly while changing positions, especially if rising from a sitting or lying position, it will reduce the likelihood of any dizziness. If you take your medicine just before going to bed, be especially careful if you need to get up during the night. For the same reason, use precaution while driving or using machinery that requires alertness or good coordination.

Do not stop taking this drug without your doctor's approval, and never stop abruptly, since this can cause a sharp rise in your blood pressure. It is advised that you gradually reduce your dosage over a two- to four-day period. Its effects may last for as long as ten days after its discontinuation.

Even though you may experience a stuffy nose, do not take any OTC medication such as nasal decongestants or cold preparations, unless you check with your doctor or pharmacist first, since many of these drugs can cause a rise in your blood pressure. Never increase the dosage of your medication without a doctor's approval. If you miss a dose, take it as soon as possible. If you are near the next scheduled dose, do not take the missed dose but resume your regular schedule. Your blood pressure will probably be closely monitored for the first four weeks to determine if the drug is effective. Notify your doctor if you are feeling depressed, experiencing frequent nightmares, or gaining weight. Women must also notify their doctor if they become pregnant while using this drug.

Since the drug may cause an upset stomach, take it with food or milk. If you are bothered by a dry mouth, sugarless gum or hard candy can give you relief.

Pregnancy
Category C (see page 103). Since the drug appears in breast milk, consult your doctor before you begin breast-feeding.

Brand Name	*Generic Name*
HYLOREL	guanadrel sulfate
	(GWAN-a-drel
	SUL-fate)

How the Drug Works
By inhibiting the release of the neurotransmitter norepine-phrine, which controls nerve impulses, it reduces the tension in the walls of the blood vessels and lowers blood pressure.

Purpose
Treatment of mild to moderate hypertension.

Dosage
Adults: Initially 5 mg taken orally daily, followed if necessary by a weekly or monthly adjustment until blood pressure is controlled; usually maintenance dose is 20 mg to 75 mg in divided doses.

Side Effects
Common: Sexual difficulties, dizziness, hypotension, drowsiness, fatigue.

Uncommon: Diarrhea or increased bowel movements, constipation, dry mouth, tremors, headaches, weight gain.

Adverse Reactions
Edema (swelling feet or ankles), chest pain, shortness of breath, coughing.

Drug Interaction
Increases the effects of other antihypertensives and sedatives. With monoamine oxidase (MAO) inhibitors, it may cause hypertension.

Overdosage
If any of the following symptoms develop, notify your physician immediately: Severe dizziness or drowsiness, fainting, cold and sweaty skin, flushed skin, severe diarrhea.

Comments
Hylorel (guanadrel sulfate) is used usually only after a "Step 1" treatment with a diuretic or beta blocker alone has not been successful. As "Step 2" medication, it's used usually with a thiazide diuretic.

Notify your doctor if you have been taking a monoamine oxidase (MAO) inhibitor within the past two weeks or suffer from depression, a peptic ulcer, or ulcerative colitis. Guanadrel should also be used cautiously if you have a history of heart disease, asthma, or heart, liver, or kidney disease.

Initially you may feel drowsy or run down with this drug, or you may experience a sudden fainting sensation during the first week of your drug therapy. It takes a while for your body to get adjusted to the lower blood pressure. If you move slowly while changing positions, especially if rising from a sitting or lying position, it will reduce the likelihood of any dizziness. Avoid strenuous exercise. Hot showers may cause a hypotensive (low blood pressure) reaction. If you take your medicine just before going to bed, be especially careful if you need to get up during the night. For the same reason, use precaution while driving or using machinery that requires alertness or good coordination.

Do not stop taking this drug without your doctor's approval, and never stop abruptly, since this can cause a sharp rise in your blood pressure. It is advised that you gradually reduce your dosage over a two- to four-day period. Its effects may last for as long as ten days after its discontinuation.

Even though you may experience a stuffy nose, do not take any OTC medication such as nasal decongestants or cold preparations, unless you check with your doctor or pharmacist first, since many of these drugs can cause a rise in your blood pressure. Never increase the dosage of your medication without a doctor's approval. If you miss a dose, take it as soon as possible. If you are near the next scheduled dose, do not take the missed dose but resume your regular schedule. Your blood pressure will probably be closely monitored for the first four weeks to determine if the drug is effective. Notify your doctor if you are feeling depressed, experiencing frequent nightmares, or gaining weight. Women must also notify their doctor if they become pregnant while using this drug.

Since the drug may cause an upset stomach, take with food or milk. If you are bothered by dry mouth, sugarless gum or hard candy can provide relief.

Pregnancy

Category B (see page 103). Since this drug appears in breast milk, it is recommended to not nurse while taking this drug.

Brand Name	*Generic Name*
ISMELIN	guanethidine monosulfate (gwa-NETH-i-deen mon-o-SUL-fate)

How the Drug Works

By inhibiting the release of the neurotransmitter norepinephrine, which controls nerve impulses, it reduces the tension in the walls of the blood vessels and lowers blood pressure.

Purpose

Treatment of moderate to severe hypertension.

Dosage
Adults: Initially 10 mg taken orally daily, followed if necessary by a weekly or monthly adjustment, until blood pressure is controlled; usually maintenance dose is 25 mg to 50 mg in divided doses.

Children: Initially 200 mcg taken orally daily, followed if necessary by increases every one to three weeks, but not to exceed a maximum dose of 1,600 mcg, or eight times initial dose.

Side Effects
Common: Dizziness, orthostatic hypotension, sexual problems, nasal congestion, diarrhea, bradycardia (slow heartbeat), drowsiness, fatigue.

Uncommon: Dry mouth, skin rash, nausea, tremors, headache, blurred vision, drooping eyelids, loss of scalp hair, depression, increased urination, weight gain.

Adverse Reactions
Edema (swelling feet or ankles), chest pain, shortness of breath.

Drug Interaction
Increases the effects of other antihypertensives and sedatives. *With MAO inhibitors,* it may cause hypertension.

Overdosage
If any of the following symptoms develop, notify your physician immediately: Severe dizziness or drowsiness, fainting, cold and sweaty skin, flushed skin, severe diarrhea.

Comments
Ismelin (guanethidine monosulfate) is used usually only after a "Step 1" treatment with a diuretic or beta blocker alone has not been successful. As "Step 2" medication, it's used usually with a thiazide diuretic.

Notify your doctor if you have been taking a monoamine

oxidase (MAO) inhibitor within the past two weeks or suffer from depression, a recent fever, a peptic ulcer, or ulcerative colitis. Ismelin should also be used cautiously if you have a history of heart, liver, or kidney disease or asthma.

Initially, you may feel drowsy or run down with this drug, or you may experience a sudden fainting sensation during the first week of your drug therapy. It takes a while for your body to get adjusted to the lower blood pressure and the full antihypertensive effects of the drug may not appear until after one to three weeks of use. If you move slowly while changing positions, especially if rising from a sitting or lying position, it will reduce the likelihood of any dizziness. Avoid strenuous exercise. Hot showers may cause a hypotensive (low blood pressure) reaction. If you take your medicine just before going to bed, be especially careful if you need to get up during the night. For the same reasons, use precaution while driving or using machinery that requires alertness or good coordination.

Do not stop taking this drug without your doctor's approval, and never stop abruptly, since this can cause a sharp rise in your blood pressure. It is advised that you gradually reduce your dosage over a two- to three-week period, especially if preparing for surgery. Its effects may last for as long as 10 days after its discontinuation.

Even though you may experience a stuffy nose, do not take any OTC medication such as nasal decongestants or cold preparations, unless you check with your doctor or pharmacist first, since many of these drugs can cause a rise in your blood pressure. Never increase the dosage of your medication without a doctor's approval. If you miss a dose, take it as soon as possible. If you are near the next scheduled dose, do not take the missed dose but resume your regular schedule. Your blood pressure will probably be closely monitored for the first four weeks to determine if the drug is effective. Notify your doctor if you are feeling depressed, experiencing frequent nightmares, or gaining weight. Women must also notify their doctor if they become pregnant while using this drug.

Since the drug may cause an upset stomach, take it with food or milk. If you are bothered by a dry mouth, sugarless gum or hard candy can give you relief.

Pregnancy

Category C (see page 103). Do not use this drug while breast-feeding.

TEN

Potassium Supplements

Brand Name	Generic Name
K-DUR	potassium chloride
K-LOR, K-LYTE/CL, KA-OCHLOR, KAON-CL, KATO, KLORVESS, KLO-TRIX, K-TAB, MICRO-K LS, EXTENCAPS, SK-POTASSIUM CHLORIDE, SLOW-K, TEN-K	potassium bicarbonate
K-LYTE, K-LYTE DS	potassium bicarbonate

The body needs the mineral potassium to perform a variety of functions: normal kidney function, passage of electrical impulses throughout the nervous system, initiation of the heartbeat and its continuation, and maintenance of the health of muscle tissue, including the heart muscle. If your body's level of potassium is excessively low or high, serious problems can result.

Hypokalemia is the condition of having low potassium. It can occur as a result of an endocrine illness, such as Cushing's Disease, but much more frequently from taking certain medications, such as diuretics, which induce elimination of potassium in the urine. Furthermore, potassium loss is more likely to occur if you are simultaneously taking other drugs such as cortisone-containing medications (steroids) with your diuretic. If, for whatever reason, hypokalemia becomes a problem, your doctor may advise you to increase your dietary intake of potassium-containing foods such as bananas and citrus fruits or switch you to another type of diuretic, such as a potassium-sparing diuretic (see page 133). Depending upon the circumstances, your doctor might even prescribe a potassium supplement. For instance, low potassium may predispose patients taking digoxin (see page 225) to develop arrhythmias. Thus, your doctor may automatically prescribe a potassium supplement if you take digoxin and a diuretic.

Potential risks. Potassium supplements can irritate the stomach. If you have a history of ulcers or stomach sensitivity, your doctor should avoid prescribing sugar-coated potassium liquid or tablets for you. Preferably, you should take potassium tablets that are *slow-release* or *sustained-release* (SR). Sustained-release (or *enteric*) supplements do not dissolve in the stomach, as other potassium preparations will, but pass through the stomach and dissolve primarily in the intestine, reducing the likelihood of causing nausea. Some preparations include a bicarbonate to "buffer" the potassium irritation.

Another concern is *hyperkalemia*, a condition of high levels of potassium in the body; it can promote dangerous heart rhythm disturbances. Hyperkalemia can result from specific drug interactions, such as with Vasotec (enalapril maleate) and a potassium-sparing diuretic. Therefore, it's important that your doctor be aware of any other medications you might be taking before prescribing potassium supplements.

Brand Name	*Generic Name*
K-DUR	potassium chloride (po-TAS-ee-um KLO-ride)
K-LOR, K-LYTE/CL, KAOCHLOR, KAON-CL, KATO, KLORVESS, KLOTRIX, K-TAB, MICRO-K LS, EXTENCAPS, SK-POTAS-SIUM CHLORIDE, SLOW-K, TEN-K	potassium bicarbonate (po-TAS-ee-um by-KAR-bo-nate)

How the Drug Works

By providing concentrations of potassium, it restores proper blood levels so as to maintain normal functions of nervous and kidney system.

Purpose

Treatment of hypokalemia.

Dosage

Adults: 40 to 100 milliequivalents taken orally daily in a minimum of two divided doses. No one dose should exceed 20 milliequivalents, which is also the recommended dose for prevention of hypokalemia.

Side Effects

Uncommon: Mild diarrhea (laxative effect).

Adverse Reactions

Common: Vomiting, nausea, intestinal distress or pain, diarrhea.
Uncommon: Chest pain, throat pain, black or red-stained stools.

Drug Interaction

With spironolactone or triamterene, may cause potassium toxicity.

Overdosage

If any of the following symptoms develop, notify your physician immediately: Listlessness, cold skin, ulceration, decreased blood pressure (hypotension), numbness of skin, heavy legs, irregular heartbeat, confusion.

Comments

Potassium chloride is a prescription medication that should be taken *only* under a doctor's supervision. Gross misuse of this medication can cause serious problems, such as ulcers, paralysis in the legs, irregular heart rhythm, convulsions, or a heart attack.

Notify your doctor if you suffer from Addison's disease (underactive adrenal gland), persistent or chronic diarrhea, heart disease, or ulcers. Your potassium blood levels may be monitored for the first four weeks to determine if proper levels are maintained. Do not chew or crush these tablets: swallow them whole. If you have difficulty swallowing this drug as a tablet, your doctor may recommend a similar drug that comes in powder form that is fruit flavored, and can be dissolved in about 6 to 8 ounces of cold water.

Take this drug following meals or with food to reduce the possibility of stomach upset or diarrhea. Never increase the dosage of your medication without a doctor's approval. If you miss a dose, and it is still within two hours of the regular schedule, take the regular dose. However, do not double your next regular dose. When preparing to discontinue its use, do not stop abruptly, especially if you are taking it with a digitalis medication.

Your doctor may advise you to eat a low-salt diet. However, do not use a salt substitute while taking this drug without first discussing it with your doctor, since many substitutes contain high levels of potassium. Also, do not take it if you are dehydrated following strenuous exercise.

Pregnancy

Category C (see page 103). The safety of this drug during breast-feeding has not been established.

Brand Name	*Generic Name*
K-LYTE Effervescent Tablets, K-LYTE DS Effervescent Tablets	potassium bicarbonate

Dosage

• Hypokalemia

Adults: One K-Lyte tab completely dissolved in 3 or 4 ounces of cold water.

Comments

This form of potassium, taken dissolved in water, is used primarily in the prevention of hypokalemia caused by thiazide diuretics. Its side effects are virtually the same as the potassium chloride preparations (see page 218).

The potassium bicarbonate tablets should be dissolved in about 6 to 8 ounces of cold water. If you do not allow them to dissolve completely or if you drink the solution too quickly, you are at greater risk of stomach or intestinal irritation. I find there are two important things in taking potassium bicarbonate: sip the drink slowly for about five minutes and take it at or following a meal; and, if you find the taste of the drink difficult to accept, ask your doctor for a product that is fruit-flavored.

Pregnancy

Category C (see page 103). The safety of this drug during breast-feeding has not been established.

ELEVEN

....

Antiarrhythmics

Brand Name	Generic Name
LANOXIN, LANOXICAPS	digoxin
NORPACE	disopyramide phosphate
PROCAN SR, PROMINE,	procainamide
PRONESTYL,	hydrochloride
PRONESTYL-SR,	
QUINAGLUTE DURA-TABS,	quinidine gluconate
DURAQUIN, QUINALAN	
CINQUIN, QUINIDEX	quinidine sulfate
EXTENTABS, QUINORA	
CARDIOQUIN	quinidine polygalac-
	turonate
TAMBOCOR	flecainide acetate
MEXITIL	mexiletine hydrochloride
CORDARONE	amiodarone

The human heart contains two sets of chambers, or pumps, through which your blood flows: the two upper chambers are the right and left atria, and the two lower chambers are the right and left ventricles. When the heart functions properly, it pumps blood constantly and consistently to all your bodily tissues. It is enabled to do this in part by an electrical impulse produced by a group of special cells in the right atrium that make up what is referred to as the "sinus node" or pacemaker, which normally fires between 50 and 100 beats per minute. This electrical charge is then transmitted to the other heart chambers to regulate the work of the two sets of pumps so they function together in a regular rhythm. When this mechanism fails—when the impulse is disrupted or blocked in any way—the heart rhythm becomes abnormal, referred to as "arrhythmia." The symptom you may have is a throbbing heartbeat or "palpitation." The sensation of an abnormal heartbeat is a single or multiple extra beat, slow or rapid fluttering of the heart.

Types of Arrhythmia

Not all abnormal heart rhythms, or arrhythmias, are the same. The most common is called "sinus tachycardia," a heartbeat that is initiated and transmitted normally, but at a rate of greater than 100 beats per minute. This accelerated rate is usually an effort to provide more blood to exercising muscles or help fight a fever; the rhythm begins and dissipates gradually. The next most common type of palpitations is an extra single beat originating in an "irritable focus" in either the atria or ventricles, producing an atrial or ventricular premature beat, which is not as effective as a normal sinus node initiated beat. If many extra beats occur in succession ("atrial or ventricular tachycardia"), you may feel your heart fluttering in your chest, you may feel light-headed, or you may even have a fainting spell if the heart rate is very rapid and an inadequate blood flow reaches your brain.

These arrhythmias begin and end abruptly. They may be associated with an underlying heart condition, such as mitral valve prolapse (MVP, see page 36), or precipitated by thyroid disease or excessive amounts of caffeine, alcohol, or stress. "Paroxysmal atrial tachycardia" is a rapid rhythm, usually 150 beats per minute, which can be associated with mitral valve prolapse, thyroid disease, or unknown causes. "Atrial flutter" occurs when the atria are firing at up to 300 beats per minute, but only half of those beats are capable of firing the ventricles. And there is "atrial fibrillation" (President Bush's arrhythmia), in which the upper chambers of the heart contract at such irregular and uncoordinated high rates that the lower chambers cannot keep up. Ventricular tachycardia and fibrillation arrhythmias are very serious because they can suddenly cause totally ineffective pumping action in the heart, dropping blood pressure and causing fainting ("syncope").

Another type of arrhythmia is called "heart block." In this case the electrical signals from the right atrium to the right and left ventricles are slowed, interrupted, or completely blocked causing the lower chambers or ventricles of the heart to beat more slowly.

Heart blocks vary in the degree of their seriousness. A first-degree heart block is symptomatic. In this instance, your heart might suffer periodic minor disruptions of its normal rhythms without causing any fuss—the arrhythmia may go undetected altogether. If it doesn't progress to a more serious level of blocking, the heart block may be detected only on an electrocardiogram. A second-degree heart block is a little more serious, usually causing irregular heartbeats. As you may note in the drug section of the book, some heart drugs cause an irregular heartbeat. If caused by a drug, your doctor will either reduce the dosage of the drug or discontinue it altogether. If symptoms develop, an artificial pacemaker may be implanted temporarily or permanently to correct the electrical impulse and restore the heartbeat to a normal rhythm (see "Artificial Pacemakers," page 111). A heart block may be detected on a routine ECG, which records 15 to 30 beats on a sheet of paper, or with a Holter monitor, which is a small, Walkman-sized box that records every single heartbeat for 24 hours. A major interruption of the heart's pumping rhythm, called a third-degree heart block, is considered serious, producing symptoms that range from fainting spells and palpitations to a loss of consciousness and convulsions.

Drugs Used in Treatment of Arrhythmias

A variety of drugs are available to treat serious arrhythmias, either to correct specific attacks of arrhythmia or to prevent future arrhythmias. In many cases the antiarrhythmic drugs your doctor prescribes can successfully correct the arrhythmia; even when this is not possible, they can reduce the frequency and severity of your problem and your symptoms.

All antiarrhythmic drugs work to correct the arrhythmia by changing the conduction of electric signals in the heart, but they don't all work the same way. One type of drug may increase or slow the pace of the signal; another may block the transmission of signals; and still another may affect the way the muscles respond, once the electrical signal is received. Different antiarrhythmic drugs are used in different circumstances, depending on the type of your arrhythmia and your response to the drug.

Potential risks: Since many of these drugs suppress normal heart function in order to correct the irregular heart rhythm, they might make you feel dizzy or breathless—some of the same problems they are designed to address. The most important risk is the potential ability of certain drugs paradoxically to increase arrhythmias rather than suppress them. One anti-arrhythmic, quinidine, can be toxic at relatively low levels in some individuals, producing a condition known as "cinchonism." As a result of such risks, doctors are especially careful to test their patients with a minimum dose before using the drug on a regular basis.

By and large, these drugs are very safe and effective in treating problems related to irregular heartbeats, and any side effects you experience will probably only be a nuisance and will just last a few days. To be on the safe side, however, notify your doctor of any side effects, and don't stop or make any change in your dosage levels or schedule. If you fail to follow exactly your doctor's instructions when taking these drugs, symptoms can develop that can range from irritating to life-threatening.

Brand Name
LANOXIN, LANOXICAPS

Generic Name
digoxin (di-JOX-in)

How the Drug Works
By increasing the availability of calcium within the heart muscle, it increases the force and efficiency of the heart's contractions and stabilizes the rate and rhythm of the heartbeat.

Purpose
Treatment of heart failure, atrial arrhythmia, atrial fibrillation and flutter, and tachycardia.

Dosage
Adults: Initially 0.5 mg to 1 mg taken orally or intravenously in divided doses for the first day as a "loading dose" to raise blood level quickly; maintenance dose is 0.125 mg to 0.5 mg.

Adults over 65 years: 0.125 mg to 0.25 mg taken orally daily as maintenance dose, depending upon general health and renal (kidney) function.

Premature infants: Beginning dose is 0.025 mg in three divided doses for first day; maintenance dose is 0.01 mg daily.

Full-term infants: Taken orally, beginning dose is 0.035 mg in divided dose for first day; taken intravenously, 0.02 mg to 0.03 mg. Maintenance dose is 0.01 mg taken orally daily in divided doses.

Children one month to two years: Taken orally, beginning dose is 0.035 mg to 0.060 mg in three divided doses for first day; intravenously, 0.03 mg to 0.05 mg. Maintenance dose is 0.01 mg to 0.02 mg taken orally daily in divided doses.

Children over two years: Taken orally, beginning dose is 0.02 mg to 0.04 mg divided dose for first day; intravenously, 0.015 mg to 0.035 mg. Maintenance dose is 0.012 mg taken orally daily in divided doses.

Side Effects
Rare: Enlargement or sensitivity of male breasts.

Adverse Reactions
Very Rare: Allergic reactions (skin rash or hives).

Signs of overdose: Loss of appetite; nausea; diarrhea; drowsiness; lethargy; changes in vision (yellow halo around lights or dark objects); confusion, especially in elderly; headache. Paradoxical increase in certain rhythm disturbance.

Drug Interaction
With adrenaline drugs, may cause irregular heart rhythms.

With cortisone-related drugs, diuretics, or thyroid preparations, may cause digitalis toxicity.

Propranolol, guanethidine, and phenytoin may increase effects of digoxin.

Antacids and laxatives may decrease effects of digoxin.

Overdosage
If any of the following symptoms develop, a physician should be notified immediately: Intestinal bleeding, anorexia, vomiting, slow pulse, delirium, convulsions.

Comments
Digoxin, introduced in 1934, was the first digitalis drug available. It is usually prescribed to treat problems of congestive heart failure, as well as an irregular or too rapid heartbeat. Although digitalis drugs are to be used *only* in the treatment of cardiac disease, on occasions digitalis has wrongly been prescribed for weight loss in people who are chronically overweight.

Notify your doctor what heart drugs you have taken and when, and whether you have a history of heart, liver, or kidney disease, or rheumatic fever. Tell your doctor if you intend to purchase an OTC medication such as cough, cold, or allergy medicine, and before taking antacids or laxatives, products that reduce absorption of digoxin.

If your pulse slows significantly or if you lose weight or experience stomach pains, nausea, blurred or yellowed vision, or depression while taking this drug, notify your doctor. Do not stop taking the drug nor increase its dosage without your doctor's approval. If you miss a scheduled dosage, do not take the missed dose and do not double the next dose.

Pregnancy
Category C (see page 103). Since the drug appears in breast milk, consult your doctor before you begin breast-feeding. Your doctor can monitor blood levels of digoxin in your body by a simple blood test.

Brand Name
NORPACE

Generic Name
disopyramide phosphate
(dye-so-PEER-a-mide
FOS-fate)

How the Drug Works
By slowing the transmission of nerve impulses to the heart, it stabilizes the rhythm of the heartbeat.

Purpose
Treatment of irregular heartbeat and tachycardia.

Dosage
Adults: 400 mg to 800 mg taken orally in divided doses. The precise amount depends upon the health of the patient (i.e., kidney, liver, or heart impairment) and body weight.

Children less than a year: 10 mg to 30 mg daily.
Children 1 to 4 years: 10 mg to 20 mg daily.
Children 4 to 12 years: 10 mg to 15 mg daily.
Children 12 to 18 years: 6 mg to 15 mg daily.

Side Effects
Common: Dry mouth, nose, and throat.
Uncommon: Blurred vision, constipation, decreased sexual ability, stomach pain.

Adverse Reactions
Urinary hesitation, chest pains, fatigue, dizziness, skin rash, muscle weakness, dry eyes, shortness of breath, unusually slow or fast heartbeat, weight gain, ankles swelling.
Rare: Signs of hypoglycemia—anxiety, chills, confusion, excessive hunger, cool skin, nervousness, cold sweats, unsteady walk.

Drug Interaction
Increases the effectiveness of warfarin and antihypertensive drugs.

With phenytoin (Dilantin), a drug taken for seizures, increases the liver metabolism of disopyramide, thereby decreasing its effectiveness.

Overdosage
If any of the following symptoms develop, a physician should be notified immediately: Increasing constipation or difficulty in urination, sharp drop in blood pressure, congestive heart failure, heart arrest.

Comments
Norpace (disopyramide phosphate), introduced in 1978, is often prescribed to patients who cannot tolerate other antiarrhythmic drugs, primarily the quinidine drugs (see page 231) or procainamide hydrochloride. Its principal therapeutic use is to correct irregular heart rhythms and rapid heartbeat. It can poten-

tially induce a hypoglycemic condition (low blood sugar). Though this is rare, if you have a history of diabetes, or kidney or liver disease, your doctor should use this drug with extreme caution. The elderly are also more susceptible to a hypoglycemic response.

Notify your doctor if you are taking any medicine whatsoever, if you have a history of prostate problems (urinary retention) or glaucoma, or if you intend to purchase an OTC medication such as cough, cold, or allergy medicine.

If your pulse slows significantly or if you lose weight or experience stomach pains, chills, sweating, or rapid heartbeat while taking this drug, notify your doctor. Do not change the dosage or discontinue the drug without your doctor's approval. Take your dosages at regular and evenly spaced intervals. If you miss a scheduled dosage, you may take it until a few hours before the next scheduled dose. Later than that, do not take the missed dose nor double the next dose. If dry mouth becomes a problem, sugarless gum or ice chips may help to relieve the dryness and moisten your mouth.

Pregnancy
Category C (see page 103). Since the drug appears in breast milk, consult your doctor before you begin breast-feeding.

Brand Name	*Generic Name*
PROCAN SR, PROMINE, PRONESTYL, PRONESTYL-SR	procainamide hydrochloride (pro-KANE-a-mide hy-dro-KLO-ride)

How the Drug Works
By slowing the transmission of nerve impulses to the heart, it stabilizes the rhythm of the heartbeat.

Purpose
Treatment of atrial fibrillation, atrial or ventricular tachycardia.

Dosage

Adults: Loading dose is 1,000 mg to 1.25 g taken orally. Then 500 mg to 1,000 mg every four to six hours.
• Ventricular tachycardia
Adults: Loading dose is 1,000 mg taken orally; average dose is 500 mg to 1000 mg every four to six hours.

Side Effects

Common: Diarrhea, poor appetite.
Uncommon: Dizziness.

Adverse Reactions

Common: Fever and chills, vomiting, joint pain, skin rash.
Rare: Hallucinations, depression, sore mouth or throat, severe bradycardia (slow heartbeat).

Drug Interaction

Effectiveness increased by other antiarrhythmic drugs.
Increases the effects of other antihypertensive drugs.

Overdosage

If any of the following symptoms develop, notify your physician immediately: Confusion, severe hypotension, fainting, fast or irregular heartbeat, stupor.

Comments

Procan SR (sustained released), introduced in 1950, is prescribed to treat various types of irregular heartbeats. Notify your doctor if you have any history of a sensitivity to procaine drugs (e.g., Novocain), if you are taking any medicine whatsoever, or if you intend to purchase an OTC medication such as cough, cold, or allergy medicine.

For about the first three months, your doctor may monitor your blood levels, especially if you are taking the sustained released form of the drug. Take your dosages exactly as prescribed, at regular and evenly spaced intervals. If you should miss a scheduled dosage by only a few hours, you may take the missed dose. Otherwise wait until the next scheduled dose and do not double the next dose.

If you notice sores in your mouth or gums, fevers, cold symptoms, or joint pains, notify your doctor. Also, the sustained release tablets have a wax core that slowly releases the drug. This nonabsorbable wax is eliminated and may be seen in your stool. The drug, however, is completely absorbed before this occurs. (A "lupus-like" reaction sometimes occurs, including skin rash, joint pain, and blood test abnormalities, but these symptoms disappear upon cessation of treatment.)

Pregnancy
Category C (see page 103). Since the drug appears in breast milk, consult your doctor before you begin breast-feeding.

Brand Name	Generic Name
QUINAGLUTE DURA-TABS, DURAQUIN, QUINALAN	quinidine gluconate (KWIN-i-deen GLOO-ko-nate)
CINQUIN, QUINIDEX EXTENTABS, QUINORA	quinidine sulfate (KWIN-i-deen SUL-fate)
CARDIOQUIN	quinidine polygalacturonate (KWIN-i-deen pol-ee-gal-ak-TYOO-ro-nate)

How the Drug Works
By slowing the transmission of electrical impulses in the heart, it stabilizes the rhythm of the heartbeat.

Purpose
Atrial and ventricular arrhythmias.

Dosage

Adults: Quinidine gluconate—one to two tabs every six hours; for maintenance of normal rhythm two tabs every 12 hours. Quinidine sulfate—300 mg to 600 mg every six hours, as needed. Quinidine polygalacturonate—one to three tabs initially, then one tab twice a day.

Side Effects

Common: Diarrhea, bitter taste, loss of appetite, nausea, vomiting, stomach cramps, rash or flushed skin.

Adverse Reactions

Fever; dizziness; ringing in the ears; change in vision; confusion; severe headache; hives, itching, or skin rash; trouble breathing.

Rare: Tachycardia (rapid heartbeat), unusual bleeding or bruising (thrombocytopenia), profound fatigue.

Drug Interaction

Increases the effectiveness of anticoagulants and antihypertensive drugs.

With phenytoin, effectiveness may be decreased.

With digoxin and propranolol, may cause serious slowing of the heart.

Overdosage

If any of the following symptoms develop, notify your physician immediately: Sharp drop in blood pressure, trouble breathing.

Comments

Quinidine, introduced in 1918 and derived from the cinchona tree, which produces quinine as well, is an old drug used to slow the heartbeat and correct irregular heart rhythm. The drug quinidine comes in three forms, with quinidine sulfate being the most active.

Notify your doctor if you have a history of overactive thyroid, angina, or heart disease, and if you are taking any medicine whatsoever, including OTC medicines such as antacids. Your doctor may periodically monitor your kidney and liver function, as well as your blood, for quinidine and potassium levels.

If your pulse is slowed significantly or if you develop a rash, fever, unusual bleeding or bruising, ringing in your ears, or, especially, diarrhea, notify your doctor. The unusual bleeding or bruising ("thrombocytopenia") is caused by the drug's tendency to decrease the number of blood platelets needed for blood clotting. (see page 241).

Depending upon the sensitivity of the patient, an overdose can occur following a single dose; hence, your doctor may give you a test dose before beginning treatment with this drug. Do not discontinue this drug without your doctor's approval and take your dosages at regular and evenly spaced intervals, preferably with meals. If you miss a scheduled dosage, you may take it up until a few hours before the next scheduled dose, but if it's later, do not take the missed dose nor double the next dose. Do not crush or chew drugs labeled "sustained release tablets."

Pregnancy
Category C (see page 103). Since the drug appears in breast milk, consult your doctor before you begin breast-feeding.

Brand Name	*Generic Name*
TAMBOCOR	flecainide acetate
	(FLEK-a-nide
	ASS-e-tate)

How the Drug Works
By slowing the transmission of nerve impulses to the heart, it stabilizes the rhythm of the heartbeat.

Purpose
Treatment of life-threatening ventricular arrhythmias, such as sustained ventricular tachycardia.

Dosage

Adults: Initially 100 mg every 12 hours, followed by increases every four days of 50 mg twice daily as needed; maximum daily dosage is usually no more than 400 mg.

Side Effects

Common: Dizziness, headaches, fatigue, tremor, blurred vision or spots before the eyes.

Uncommon: Nausea or vomiting, constipation, anxiety, depression.

Adverse Reactions

New or aggravated heart rhythm disturbances (especially at higher doses), shortness of breath ("bronchospasm") or difficulty getting enough air ("dyspnea"), chest pain, edema, urinary retention.

Drug Interaction

Increases the effectiveness of antihypertensive drugs such as propranolol and digoxin.

Levels may be increased by Tagamet.

Effectiveness may be decreased by phenytoin.

Overdosage

If any of the following symptoms develop, notify your physician immediately: Sharp drop in blood pressure, trouble breathing.

Comments

Tambocor (flecainide acetate) is used to treat life-threatening heart rhythm disturbances. Its most serious adverse reaction is "pro-arrhythmia": It can produce or worsen heart rhythm disturbances. These effects are more likely to occur when the dose level of the drug is high and in patients with a history of heart disease. Hence, under no circumstances should you change the dose of this drug without the supervision of your doctor.

Notify your doctor if you have a history of heart disease, or if you are taking any medicine whatsoever, including OTC medicines. Your doctor may periodically monitor your kidney and liver function as well as your blood for potassium levels, for high or low potassium levels can alter effectiveness of this drug.

If you miss a scheduled dosage by six hours or less, take it as soon as possible. Use precaution while driving or using machinery that requires alertness or good coordination.

Pregnancy
Category C (see page 103).

Brand Name	*Generic Name*
MEXITIL	mexiletine hydrochloride
	(mex-IL-e-teen
	hy-dro-KLO-ride)

How the Drug Works
By slowing the transmission of nerve impulses to the heart, it stabilizes the rhythm of the heartbeat.

Purpose
Treatment of ventricular arrhythmias.

Dosage
Adults: For rapid control, 400 mg taken orally followed by 200 mg eight hours later. If rapid control is not crucial, 200 mg every eight hours initially, followed by an upward or downward adjustment of 50 mg to 100 mg. Increase to 300 mg every eight hours if response is not satisfactory. Depending upon toleration, drug can be taken at 400 mg every eight hours, but changes in dosages should be made at intervals of two to three days.

Side Effects

Common: Nausea, nervousness, heartburn, dizziness, tremors, shakiness or difficult walking, constipation, changes in sleeping habits, blurred vision.

Less common: Headache, skin rash, diarrhea, confusion, changes in appetite, ringing in ears, unusual tiredness, slurred speech, depression, numbness of fingers or feet, urinary hesitations.

Adverse Reactions

Heart palpitations, chest pain, irregular heartbeat.

Rare: Fever, chills, sore throat, seizures, unusual bleeding or bruising.

Drug Interaction

With Phenytoin, rifampin, and phenobarbital, effectiveness may be decreased.

With cemetidine, blood levels are increased.

Overdosage

If any of the following symptoms develop, a physician should be notified immediately: Excessive hypotension, seizures.

Comments

Mexitil (mexilitine hydrochloride) is used to correct or prevent irregular heartbeats by slowing the nerve impulses to the heart, which makes the heart muscle less sensitive.

For the drug to be most effective, you should have a constant amount in your blood, which is why your doctor will probably have you take the drug at regular eight-hour intervals around the clock. Your doctor may place you on a 12-hour schedule if you do not experience any diminished effects, which means you can take the drug with your morning and evening meals. Do not discontinue this drug without your doctor's approval. If you miss a dose, take it as soon as possible, but if more than four hours have lapsed in your eight-hour schedule, skip the missed dose and go back to your regular schedule. At no time should you double your dose.

To reduce possible stomach irritation, the drug should be taken with food or an antacid; but avoid antacids with a magnesium or aluminum base, as they may decrease the rate of the drug's absorption. If you are taking digoxin (see page 225) with this drug, the antacid may also reduce effectiveness.

Report to your doctor any signs of tremors in your hands and dizziness, since this may indicate that your blood levels are too high.

Pregnancy

Category C (see page 103). Since the drug appears in breast milk, consult your doctor before you begin breast-feeding.

Brand Name	*Generic Name*
CORDARONE	Amiodarone

How the Drug Works

By slowing transmission of electrical impulses through the heart and inhibiting sympathetic nerve stimulation, it stabilizes the rhythm of the heartbeat.

Purpose

Treatment of serious atrial or ventricular arrhythmias.

Dosage

Loading dose: 800 to 1600 mg a day for 1 to 3 weeks, then reduced to 600 to 800 mg a day for 1 month. Maintenance dosage is usually 200–400 mg once or twice a day taken with meals.

Side Effects

Common: Photosensitivity, nausea and vomiting.

Less common: Fatigue, tremors, tingling of fingers, walking imbalance, blurred vision.

Adverse Reactions

Pulmonary toxicity manifested by progressive shortness of breath, cough, heart palpitations, irregular heartbeat, elevation of liver enzymes, profound slowing or fatigue (hypothyroidism).

Drug Interaction:

Increases effects of digoxin, Coumadin, Quinidine, Procainamide.

Overdose:

Profound hypotension.

Comments:

Cordarone (amiodarone) is used to correct or prevent irregular heartbeats by slowing the electrical impulses in the heart and inhibiting nerve stimulation to the heart. Because of its slow absorption into the body, Cordarone may take up to several weeks to be effective. Therefore, very high doses are used to initiate therapy over the course of one week in the hospital. Once the drug is stopped, it remains in your body for up to one year, continuing your risk for side effects, such as photosensitivity. Because of its side effects, cordarone is usually one of the last antiarrhythmic drugs utilized.

Pregnancy:
Category C (see page 103).

TWELVE

Blood-Related Drugs

ANTICOAGULANT AGENTS

Brand Name	*Generic Name*
COUMADIN	warfarin sodium
HEPARIN, LIQUAEMIN	heparin sodium

THROMBOLYTIC AGENTS

Brand Name	*Generic Name*
KABIKINASE, STREPTASE	streptokinase
ACTIVASE	alteplase, recombinant

HEMORHEOLOGIC AGENTS

Brand Name	*Generic Name*
TRENTAL	pentoxifylline

ANTIPLATELET AGENTS

Brand Name	*Generic Name*
PERSANTINE, PYRIDAMOLE	dipyridamole
BUFFERIN and many other aspirin-containing medications	acetylsalicylic acid

Coagulation

The ability for your blood to coagulate, or form clots, is absolutely critical to your recovery from an injury or surgery or even a minor cut, because when bleeding occurs the clotting of the blood seals the wound or break in the blood vessel. An inability to form blood clots when needed is relatively rare; the tendency to form clots when there is no need for them is a far more common and serious problem, called thrombosis. The total obstruction of a vein or artery is called an *occlusion*.

The clotting mechanism in your blood begins when blood platelets gather at the site of a wound to form a plug and close the openings in the blood vessels. These cells also aid in the production of a filamentlike protein, fibrin. The fine weblike filaments of fibrin hold together the white and red cells, as well as the sticky platelets, to coagulate or clot.

The formation of fibrin depends upon the presence of plasma proteins, or clotting factors. When these proteins are absent or ineffective, an inherited disease, referred to as hemophilia, exists. Because fibrin cannot be formed and blood clotting is impaired or fails, a hemophiliac may suffer from deep internal bleeding, producing symptoms such as painful joints, blood in the urine or stool, excessive bruising, and severe nosebleeds. People with hemophilia are not usually treated with drugs, although in certain circumstances, such as during necessary surgery, they are given a concentrated form of the missing clotting factor to help promote clotting and stop the bleeding.

The tendency to bleed is not, however, always an inherited condition. Many people develop a blood disorder that impairs their blood clotting; the most common cause of impaired clotting is excessive aspirin ingestion. Patients with liver disease or who chronically abuse alcohol can impair coagulation, and a gross vitamin K deficiency may also result in a bleeding disorder because the vitamin is essential to produce an enzyme that leads to the conversion and production of the protein fibrin. Since the vitamin is absorbed through the intestine with the help of fats, someone suffering from a fat absorption disorder could develop a vitamin K deficiency.

For heart disease patients and their doctors, however, the emphasis is on eliminating and preventing blood clots from forming in the circulatory system. Clots can form when blood flow is slowed or disturbed, often because of the presence of fatty deposits that form on the walls of the blood vessel, a condition referred to as atherosclerosis. The blood clot not only disrupts the flow of blood where it is formed, but can become dislodged and move through the blood system. This poses a highly dangerous situation since it can eventually become lodged in a vessel that supplies blood to a vital organ, such as your heart or brain. If the lodged blood clot effectively cuts off the supply of a fresh blood, the cells of the organ will begin to die, causing a heart attack or stroke.

Drugs

Drugs that treat the problem of blood clots, by dissolving or preventing them, fall into three general categories: anticoagulants, thrombolytics, and antiplatelets.

Anticoagulants. Anticoagulants, which reduce the production of fibrin, the filamentlike protein on which clotting depends, generally are used to prevent clots from forming, although some of these drugs also are prescribed to prevent a clot from breaking loose. Some anticoagulants are given intravenously, others orally. The intravenous anticoagulant is fast acting, whereas oral anticoagulants take effect after a day or two. The most common intravenous anticoagulant, Heparin, is most often used following surgery to prevent a blood clot from forming on an artificial heart valve or in a vein in your leg. Oral anticoagulants, which are more convenient to take at home, are used to prevent clots from forming and often are given following a hospital administration of Heparin.

Thrombolytics. Thrombolytic drugs, usually hospital administered, work to break up clots that have already formed, by raising the level of an enzyme in the blood that breaks down the existing fibrin. These drugs are administered both intravenously and directly into the blocked artery. They are primarily utilized during a heart attack to promote dissolution of the blood clot blocking a vital coronary artery.

Antiplatelets. Antiplatelet drugs reduce the stickiness of blood platelets, which reduces their ability to form clots. Of all the drugs that affect blood clotting, these drugs have the fewest side effects and risks; if administered properly, they can be taken on a daily basis over a period of months or even years. These drugs are especially valuable following heart surgery, to prevent clots from forming in blood vessel grafts. Aspirin, known primarily as an analgesic or pain killer, is probably the most widely used antiplatelet drug. Many of my patients who have suffered intestinal distress with aspirin use in the past have been able to successfully tolerate aspirin as an antiplatelet, since it is effective at much lower doses, and consequently is less likely to cause any side effects, than other anticoagulants.

Potential Risks

Drugs that reduce blood clotting can also produce excessive bleeding, especially if the dose is not correct. Signs of bleeding are blood in the urine (red or dark urine) or rectum (black or red stool), easy bruising, or heavy menstrual bleeding.

Because these particular drugs interact with so many other drugs, it is important that you tell your doctor if you are taking any other drugs, prescription or nonprescription. For example, the regular use of aspirin can increase the anticoagulating potential of a drug and cause excessive bleeding. Analgesic products such as Indocin, Nuprin, or Motrin may also increase the effects of an anticoagulant such as Coumadin.

It is also advised that you do not drink alcohol with these drugs or change your diet drastically, and contact your doctor if you are to have serious dental work or elective surgery.

ANTICOAGULANT AGENTS

Brand Name
COUMADIN

Generic Name
warfarin sodium (WAR-far-in SO-dee-am)

How the Drug Works
By blocking the action of vitamin K, it disrupts the production of essential blood-clotting factors, which reduces the likelihood of clots forming in the blood.

Purpose
Treatment of venous thrombosis, pulmonary (in a vessel carrying blood to or from the lungs) embolism, atrial fibrillation (with embolism). Prevention of embolisms following a heart attack.

Dosage
Adults: Initially 10 mg taken orally for two to four days, followed by doses of 2 mg to 10 mg daily for maintenance.

Side Effects
Common: Bloated stomach or gas, nausea, vomiting.
Uncommon: Hair loss, flushed skin, blurred vision, loss of appetite.

Adverse Reactions
Painful urination, cloudy or dark urine, decrease in amount of urine; sores in mouth or throat; weight gain; fatigue; yellowing eyes or skin; bleeding (*signs of bleeding*: bleeding gums, nose bleeds, bruising, heavy menstrual bleeding, stomach pain or swelling, blood in the urine, coughing up blood, dizziness, joint pain, vomiting blood—which looks like coffee grounds).

Drug Interaction

Many drug interactions, with thiazide diuretics, barbiturates, antibiotics, laxatives, oral contraceptives, aspirin, and others.

Effectiveness may be increased with nonsteroidal anti-inflammatory analgesic products such as indomethacin (Indocin) or ibuprofen (Nuprin and Motrin).

Overdosage

If any of the following symptoms develop, notify your physician immediately: Signs of internal bleeding, such as vomiting blood and bloody stools and urine.

Comments

Coumadin (warfarin sodium), introduced in 1954, is an anticoagulant popularly though incorrectly referred to as a "blood thinner." Although the drug reduces the likelihood of blood clot formation by preventing the liver from making blood-clotting substances, it will not dissolve clots already formed or heal any vascular damage produced by blood clots.

Perhaps few other drugs interact with so many others as do anticoagulants. Hence, it is important that you tell your doctor if you are taking any other drugs, prescription or nonprescription. The regular use of aspirin can increase the anticoagulating potential of warfarin sodium and cause excessive bleeding in some patients, so it is important to check other preparations, such as cough capsules, as they may contain aspirin. Analgesic products such as Indocin, Nuprin, or Motrin may also increase the effects or the pro-time of the Coumadin (see page 69); therefore their use must be watched carefully. Tell your doctor if you take these medications.

This drug requires that you pay attention to your intake of vitamin K (from the German word *Koagulation*). Vitamin K is necessary to the formation of blood-clotting substances, and excessive intake of vitamin K can actually blunt the effectiveness of the Coumadin taken to block vitamin K's action. So while taking

Coumadin do not eat excessively large amounts of foods rich in vitamin K, such as cabbage, cauliflower, spinach, and other leafy green vegetables. Eat only moderate amounts and basically the same amount each day, as any significant change in your diet could affect the drug's effectiveness. Vitamin E supplements should not be taken while using this drug since they reduce the absorption of vitamin K and could cause bleeding.

Take the drug on an empty stomach because food slows its absorption, and take it at the same time each day. If you miss a dose, take it as soon as possible. But if you do not remember until the next day, skip the missed dose and go back to your regular schedule. Do not double your dose for any reason, as it may cause internal bleeding. Finally, do not stop the drug without informing your doctor.

Notify your doctor if you experience any unusual bleeding or bruising including heavy menstrual bleeding, red or dark brown urine, black or tarry stools, or diarrhea. Do not change specific-name-brands of this drug without consulting your doctor, as they are not all the same.

Pregnancy

Category D (see page 103). Since the drug appears in breast milk, this drug should not be used if you are breast-feeding.

Brand Name	*Generic Name*
HEPARIN, LIQUAEMIN	heparin sodium
	(HEP-a-rin SO-dee-am)

How the Drug Works

By blocking the action of the enzyme thrombin, it prevents the conversion of the protein fibrinogen into fibrin, thereby reducing the likelihood of clots forming in the blood.

Purpose

Prevention and treatment of venous thrombosis, pulmonary embolism, atrial fibrillation (with embolism). Prevention of embolisms following a heart attack.

Dosage

Adults: Administered intravenously or subcutaneously in different dosages.

Side Effects

Chest pain, fever or chills, blood blister at injection site, runny nose, rash or itchy skin, shortness of breath, pains in arms or legs.

All the symptoms resulting from the use of this drug, whether considered a side effect or an adverse reaction, should be reported to your doctor or nurse.

Adverse Reactions

Signs of internal bleeding: Bleeding gums, nosebleeds, bruising, heavy menstrual bleeding, stomach pain or swelling, blood in the urine, coughing up blood, dizziness, joint pain, vomiting blood— which looks like coffee grounds.

Drug Interaction

Increases risk of bleeding with anticoagulants, aspirin, thrombolytic agents, among others.

Anticoagulant effects impaired with digitalis, tetracyclines, antihistamines.

Overdosage

If any of the following symptoms develop, notify your physician immediately: Signs of internal bleeding, such as vomiting blood, and bloody stools and urine.

Comments

Since Heparin (heparin sodium) is an extremely fast-acting anticoagulant that is administered by injection, it is usually used in an emergency in a hospital setting to help prevent clots from forming or getting bigger. The drug is also regularly used to prevent blood clots forming in veins, a condition called phlebitis, or their being dislodged and carried through the bloodstream into the lungs.

Pregnancy
Category C (see page 103).

THROMBOLYTIC AGENTS

Brand Name   *Generic Name*
KABIKINASE, STREPTASE   streptokinase
                             (strep-to-KY-nase)

How the Drug Works
By increasing the action of an enzyme in the blood called plasmin, the drug breaks up the strands of fibrin that hold the blood platelets together in a clot.

Purpose
Treatment of myocardial infarction, pulmonary embolism, deep vein and arterial thrombosis or embolism.

Dosage
• Myocardial infarction
   Adults: Initially 1.5 million international units (IU) given intravenously in the course of one hour; alternatively, 20,000 IU delivered directly into the thrombosed artery, followed by 2,000 IU for 60 minutes.
• Pulmonary embolism:
   Adults: Initially 250,000 IU intravenously over 30 minutes, followed by 100,000 IU for 24 hours.
• Deep vein and arterial thrombosis or embolism
   Adults: Initially 250,000 IU intravenously over 30 minutes,

followed by 100,000 IU for 72 hours for deep vein thrombosis or 24 to 72 hours for arterial thrombosis or embolism.

Side Effects

Virtually any side effects produced by the drug are considered adverse and should be reported to your nurse or doctor.

Adverse Reactions

Bleeding from cuts or puncture site of injection, fever, slow or irregular heartbeat.

Rare: Swelling around the eyes, rash or redness of skin, headache, nausea, muscle pain, shortness of breath.

Signs of internal bleeding: Nosebleeds, easy bruising, heavy menstrual bleeding, stomach pain or swelling, blood in the urine, constipation, black and tarry stool, coughing up blood, dizziness, joint pain, severe headaches, vomiting blood—which looks like coffee grounds.

Drug Interaction

May cause increased bleeding with anticoagulants, aspirin, indomethacin, and other drugs that affect blood platelet activity.

Overdosage

If any of the following symptoms develop, notify your physician immediately: Signs of internal bleeding, such as vomiting blood, and bloody stools and urine.

Comments

Streptokinase is a thrombolytic agent—it breaks up or dissolves blood clots—and is used only in a hospital. Since it is administered intravenously and excessive bleeding is a potential effect, you will be closely monitored, probably every half hour or so, for about eight hours, and then far less frequently.

Pregnancy

Category C (see page 103). Since the drug appears in breast milk, consult your doctor before you begin breast-feeding.

Brand Name	Generic Name
ACTIVASE	alteplase, recombinant

How the Drug Works
By increasing the action of an enzyme in the blood called plasmin, the drug breaks up the strands of fibrin that hold the blood platelets together in a clot.

Purpose
Treatment of acute myocardial infarction.

Dosage
Adults: 60 mg in first hour: 6 mg to 10 mg intravenously for first minute or two and the remainder 50 mg to 54 mg intravenously, followed by 40 mg over the next two hours by I.V. infusion. (Dosages will be affected by your body weight.)

Side Effects
Virtually any effects produced by the drug are considered adverse and should be reported to your nurse or doctor.

Adverse Reactions
Bleeding from cuts or puncture site of injection, fever, slow or irregular heartbeat.

Rare: Swelling around the eyes, rash or redness of skin, headache, nausea, muscle pain, shortness of breath, internal bleeding (rare).

Signs of Internal Bleeding: nosebleeds, easy bruising, heavy menstrual bleeding, stomach pain or swelling, blood in the urine, constipation, black and tarry stool, coughing up blood, dizziness, joint pain, severe headaches, vomiting blood—which looks like coffee grounds.

Drug Interaction

May cause increased bleeding with anticoagulants, or aspirin, indomethacin, and other drugs that affect blood platelet activity.

Overdosage

If any of the following symptoms develop, notify your physician immediately: Signs of internal bleeding, such as vomiting blood, and bloody stools and urine.

Comments

Activase (recombinant alteplase) is a thrombolytic agent—it breaks up blood clots—and like streptokinase is used only in a hospital, often in emergencies. Also referred to as a tissue-type plasminogen activator (TPA), it is infused directly into the vein or artery to quickly dissolve a clot and restore blood flow to the heart muscle.

In some instances it will also be prescribed for treatment of blood clots in the lungs, and angina. Since it is administered intravenously and excessive bleeding is a potential effect, you will be closely monitored, probably every half hour or so, for about eight hours and then far less frequently.

Pregnancy

Category C (see page 103). Since the drug appears in breast milk, consult your doctor before you begin breast-feeding.

HEMORHEOLOGIC AGENTS

Brand Name
TRENTAL

Generic Name
pentoxifylline
(pen-tox-IF-i-lin)

How the Drug Works

By increasing the flexibility of red blood cells and lowering the viscosity or stickiness of the blood, it increases the flow of blood.

Purpose

Intermittent claudication (inadequate blood flow to legs)

Dosage

Adults: Initially 400 mg three times daily for at least eight weeks. Adjustments downward may be necessary if digestive or neurological reactions occur.

Side Effects

Uncommon: Dizziness, nausea, upset stomach, headache.

Adverse Reactions

Rare: Chest pain, hypotension, irregular heartbeat.

Drug Interaction

Increases effects of antihypertensives.

Overdosage

If any of the following symptoms develop, a physician should be notified immediately: Flushing, dizziness, faintness, drowsiness, restlessness, fever, convulsions, seizures.

Comments

Trental (pentoxifylline), a relatively new drug, is used to treat peripheral vascular disease, especially the symptoms of leg pain or cramps caused by poor circulation. By increasing the flexibility of the oxygen-carrying red blood cells, sometimes referred to as "thinning the blood," the drug allows the cells to flow through the smallest capillaries, especially those in your fingers or eyes. Doctors use pentoxifylline to treat circulatory problems related to diabetes, leg ulcers, strokes, circulation problems of the eyes or hands, high-altitude sickness, and hearing problems.

Relief from your leg cramps or pains may not occur immediately: Symptoms may continue for the first two to four weeks of drug use. Your doctor will have you take this drug for a minimum of eight weeks, during which time you are not to stop taking it without your doctor's approval. It can upset your stomach, so don't crush or chew the tablet, but swallow it whole, and take it with food or your meals. If you miss a dose, take it as soon as possible. But if it is almost time for the next dose, skip the missed dose and go back to your regular schedule. Do not double your dose.

Any intestinal or neurological problems such as restlessness should be reported to your doctor. To reduce these symptoms, your doctor may reduce the dosage or discontinue the drug. Smoking is always a serious threat to your health; it can cause your blood vessels to constrict and reduce the effectiveness of pentoxifylline.

Pregnancy

Category C (see page 103). Since the drug appears in breast milk, consult your doctor before you begin breast-feeding.

ANTIPLATELET AGENTS

Brand Name
PERSANTINE,
   PYRIDAMOLE

Generic Name
dipyridamole
   (dy-peer-ID-a-mole)

How the Drug Works

By widening the small arteries and preventing blood platelets from coagulating, it reduces clotting and eases blood flow. The drug is particularly effective in combination with warfarin (page 244) to reduce clot formation on metal heart valves.

Purpose

Reduction of blood platelet adhesion, treatment of transient ischemic attack (temporary anemia due to obstruction of circulation).

Dosage

• Blood platelet adhesion
    Adults: 75 mg to 100 mg taken orally four times daily.
• Transient ischemic attack
    Adults: 400 mg to 800 mg taken orally in divided doses.

Side Effects

Uncommon: Dizziness, stomach cramps, headache, flushing, nausea, weakness.

Adverse Reactions

Rare: Tightness in the chest, anginalike pains.

Drug Interaction

Persantine does not influence the pro-time (PT) in patients taking warfarin (page 244).

Overdosage

If any of the following symptoms develop, notify your physician immediately: Weak or rapid pulse, cold or clammy skin, collapse.

Comments

Dipyridamole's antiplatelet action prevents blood platelets from clumping together, and the drug is often prescribed with warfarin sodium (Coumadin) or aspirin following heart valve surgery. Because it also acts as a vasodilator, some doctors prescribe it, along with aspirin, to treat the pain of angina and to prevent heart attacks.

Notify your doctor if you are taking any other drugs, including OTC products such as aspirin. It is preferable to take the drug with a full glass of water about an hour or two before your meal for maximum absorption; but if you experience an upset stomach, take it with milk or with your meals.

Do not stop taking the drug without your doctor's approval. If you miss a dose, take it as soon as possible, unless it is within four hours of your next dose; then, skip the missed dose and resume your regular schedule. Do not double your dose. Do not change your specific-name-brand of dipyridamole without consulting your doctor; all brands are not the same or equally effective.

Pregnancy
Category C (see page 103). Since the drug appears in breast milk, consult your doctor before you begin breast-feeding.

Brand Name	*Generic Name*
BUFFERIN and many other aspirin-containing medications	acetylsalicylic (a-SEE-ti-sal-i-SIL-ic) acid (aspirin)

How the Drug Works
By blocking the production of prostaglandin, a fatty acid, it reduces the ability of the blood to form clots.

Purpose
Prevention of strokes and myocardial infarction.

Dosage
Adults: one tab once daily.

Side Effects
Uncommon: Heartburn.

Adverse Reactions

Rare: Nausea, vomiting, stomach pain, rash or hives, unusual fatigue.

Drug Interaction

Increases effects of anticoagulants.
Decreases effects of tetracycline and spironolactone.

Overdosage

If any of the following symptoms develop, a physician should be notified immediately: Nausea, vomiting, ringing in the ears, thirst, headache, diarrhea, tachycardia, hemorrhage, convulsions.

Comments

Bufferin, or aspirin, is a nonprescription nonnarcotic analgesic that has been used since 1899 for the relief of pain, fever, and the symptoms of arthritis. Recently, the anticoagulant properties of aspirin-based products have been recommended as a preventative for people who have suffered a heart attack or who have a relatively high-risk profile (see page 88).

Pregnancy

Category B (see page 103).

THIRTEEN

Antihyperlipidemics

Brand Name	Generic Name
QUESTRAN	cholestyramine
COLESTID	colestipol
ATROMID-S	clofibrate
LOPID	gemfibrozil
MEVACOR	lovastatin
NICOLAR	niacin or
	nicotinic acid
LORELCO	probucol
CHOLOXIN	dextrothyroxine

Your blood contains several kinds of fats, or lipids, all of which are necessary to growth and good health (see page 33). If certain lipids, often called unsaturated fats, reach excessive levels, they can cause atherosclerosis. Atherosclerosis is a buildup of fatty deposits, or atheromas, on the wall of the blood vessel that poses a major risk of heart disease. Atherosclerosis not only narrows the passageway of blood vessels, increasing blood pressure, but it also disrupts the flow of blood, which can lead to the formation of blood clots.

Hyperlipidemia, or excessive fat in the blood, is usually the result of diet: We eat too many fatty foods. Our body probably produces enough cholesterol to meet all our needs, independent of our dietary intake. This is true of other lipids as well. Consequently, adults probably need very little fat in their daily diets. This means that most people with high blood fat levels can reduce them by making changes in their diets.

For people who are unable to reduce their blood fat to acceptable levels by diet alone, who may have an enzyme deficiency preventing proper metabolism of fats, we have lipid-lowering, or antihyperlipidemic, drugs—different specific drugs, depending upon the kind of fat involved. Your doctor might also recommend a therapy of lipid-lowering drugs if you were suffering from a circulatory disorder or if you were at risk for coronary heart disease.

Almost any treatment to prevent the formation of fatty deposits is likely to include a variety of strategies beyond simply taking a drug. For example, you probably will be placed on a regimen to reduce other relevant risks such as smoking or obesity, and be advised to exercise regularly.

Antihyperlipidemic drugs can reduce the level of blood fat in two ways: by blocking the absorption of fat into the bloodstream or preventing the production of fats in the liver.

Drugs that act on the liver, such as clofibrate (see page 263) and gemfibrozil (see page 265), reduce the fats in the blood by preventing the conversion of fatty acids into lipids. Normally, an enzyme in the liver combines with these fatty acids to form lipids. But certain drugs are capable of changing the activity of the enzyme to reduce or prevent the production of these lipids.

Another means by which drugs can reduce blood fat levels involves their absorption. One normal liver function is to produce bile salts, a compound containing certain types of fats, primarily cholesterol, which are needed in the routine digestion of our food. Drugs such as cholestyramine (see page 259) and colestipol (see page 261), reduce cholesterol levels by blocking the reabsorption of these cholesterol-containing bile salts from the intestine into the bloodstream after they have helped in digestion.

It is important to understand that however effective these drugs can be in lowering fat levels in the blood, they do not remove lipid deposits, nor do they correct the underlying problem that may have caused the hyperlipidemia. In addition, for many of these drugs to work effectively, you will need to maintain a special diet that restricts your cholesterol and fat intake. Despite these caveats, these drugs have proved to be capable of lowering lipid levels in most cases and are therefore valuable tools in reducing the risk or development of atherosclerosis.

Potential risks: Most lipid-lowering drugs are considered relatively safe. Drugs that reduce cholesterol levels by blocking the reabsorption of bile salts from the intestine remain primarily in the intestine or bowel and are excreted with other waste products. Although they produce the fewest side effects, there is the risk that they might bar the absorption of certain other foods and vitamins, especially the fat-soluble vitamins A, D, E, and K. Drugs that act on the liver can produce more persistent side effects, such as nausea or diarrhea, because the liver ends up producing more bile salts, which can cause stomach upset for some people. One drug, clofibrate, bears additional risks in that it can potentially cause gallstones or increase the risk of heart disease. But even these drugs produce few serious side effects and can be taken with little disruption to your normal life.

Brand Name	Generic Name
QUESTRAN	cholestyramine
	(ko-les-TEER-a-meen)

How the Drug Works

By binding bile acids and cholesterol in the intestine and preventing their reabsorption, it reduces the amount of cholesterol reabsorbed into the bloodstream.

Purpose
Treatment of hypercholesterolemia and coronary artery disease.

Dosage
Adults: 4 grams or a level scoopful one to six times a day.

Side Effects
Common: Constipation.
Less Common: Diarrhea, belching, bloating, indigestion, stomach pain, nausea.

Adverse Reactions
Skin rash, black and tarry stools.
Rare: Weight loss.

Drug Interaction
Decreases the effectiveness of anticoagulants, beta blockers, steroids, digitalis, thiazide diuretics, and thyroid hormones.

Overdosage
If any of the following symptoms develop, notify your physician immediately: Chronic constipation.

Comments
Questran (cholestyramine) is used to lower cholesterol levels by increasing the removal of fat-containing bile acids from the bowel. The drug attaches itself to the bile acids in the intestine, causing them to be excreted with the body's other waste products. Bile acids are needed for digestion, so as the body begins to lose bile acids because of the action of the drug, the liver converts more cholesterol from the blood to bile acids. This process results in lower levels of cholesterol in the blood.

Because of their binding properties, this drug and Colestid (colestipol) are occasionally prescribed in cases of digitalis toxicity. Since cholestyramine is not absorbed into the bloodstream, it produces few side effects. However, many people experience constipation, and some others suffer from gas or heartburn. If constipation develops, drink more fluids and eat a high-fiber diet. If necessary, your doctor may prescribe a stool softener, reduce the dosage of your drug, or switch you to another. If any intestinal symptoms persist, or if you experience bleeding from the gums or rectum, notify your doctor.

Take cholestyramine before your full meals. If you are taking other medications, take them one hour before or at least four hours after cholestyramine. It is best to mix the powder with 6 ounces of water or a noncarbonated drink (carbonation will make the drug very foamy), although some people choose to mix it with a light meal of only cereal or soup.

If you miss a dose, take it as soon as possible, but if it is almost time for the next dose, skip the missed dose and return to your normal schedule. Do not take a double dose. While taking this drug, your doctor may also require that you take an all-purpose vitamin pill that contains vitamins A, D, and K, and folic acid.

Pregnancy

Category C (see page 103). Since the drug appears in breast milk, consult your doctor before you begin breast-feeding.

Brand Name
COLESTID

Generic Name
colestipol
(ko-LES-ti-pole)

How the Drug Works

By binding bile acids and cholesterol in the intestine and preventing their reabsorption, it reduces the amount of cholesterol reabsorbed into the bloodstream.

Purpose

Treatment of hypercholesterolemia.

Dosage
Adults: 15 grams to 30 grams daily in divided doses.

Side Effects
Common: Constipation.
Less common: Belching, indigestion, nausea, diarrhea, stomach pain.

Adverse Reactions
Black and tarry stools, severe stomach pain and vomiting.
Rare: Weight loss.

Drug Interaction
Decreases the effectiveness of anticoagulants, beta blockers, steroids, digitalis, thiazide diuretics, and thyroid hormones.

Overdosage
If any of the following symptoms develop, notify your physician immediately: Chronic constipation.

Comments
Like Questran (see page 259), Colestid (colestipol) is a drug used to lower cholesterol levels by increasing the removal of fat-containing bile acids from the bowel. The drug attaches itself to the bile acids in the intestine and causes them to be excreted with the other waste products of the body. Bile acids are needed for digestion, so as the body begins to lose bile acids because of the action of the drug, the liver converts more cholesterol from the blood to bile acids. This process results in lower levels of cholesterol in the blood.

Because of their binding properties, this drug and Questran (cholestyramine) are occasionally prescribed in cases of digitalis toxicity. Since the drug is not absorbed into the bloodstream, it produces few side effects, though many people experience constipation, and some suffer from gas or heartburn. If constipa-

tion develops, drink more fluids and eat a high-fiber diet. If necessary, your doctor may prescribe a stool softener, reduce the dosage
of your drug, or switch you to another. If intestinal symptoms
persist, or if you experience bleeding from the gums or rectum,
notify your doctor.

Take Colestid before or with your meals. Take any other medications one hour before or at least four hours after you take this
drug. It is best to mix the powder with 3 ounces of milk, juice, or
water, although some people choose to mix it with their cereal or
soup. If some of the drug sticks to the sides of the glass, mix with
more water and drink it.

If you miss a dose, take it as soon as possible, but if it is almost time for the next dose, skip the missed dose and return to
your normal schedule. Do not take a double dose. While taking
this drug, your doctor may also require that you take an all-
purpose vitamin pill that contains vitamins A, D, and K, and
folic acid.

Pregnancy
Category C (see page 103). Since the drug appears in breast
milk, consult your doctor before you begin breast-feeding.

Brand Name   *Generic Name*
ATROMID-S   clofibrate (klo-FY-brate)

How the Drug Works
By inhibiting the production of cholesterol and triglycerides
(fatlike substances) in the liver, it reduces fat blood levels.

Purpose
Treatment of hypercholesterolemia (Type III) and hypertriglyceridemia (Types IV and V).

Dosage

Adults: 2 g daily in divided doses, although some patients may find lower doses equally effective.

Side Effects

Common: Diarrhea, nausea.

Less common: Gas, heartburn, or stomach upset; vomiting; weight gain; flulike symptoms; difficult urination; headache; fatigue; itching skin.

Adverse Reactions

Rare: Anginalike pain, irregular heartbeat, shortness of breath, gallstones, swelling of feet or legs (edema), blood in the urine.

Drug Interaction

Increases the effectiveness of oral anticoagulants and antidiabetic medications, including furosemide.

Effectiveness may be decreased by oral contraceptives.

Overdosage

If any of the following symptoms develop, notify your physician immediately: Adverse reactions, including headaches, muscular pain, and weakness.

Comments

Atromid-S (clofibrate), introduced in 1967, is used to lower triglyceride and cholesterol levels, but only after diet and other therapies have failed. It is to be used cautiously because it can cause the nausea and aching muscles of a flu and can cause serious side effects, such as gallstones, heart disease, and cancer. If you experience these symptoms, report them to your doctor immediately. While taking the drug, your urine and blood levels will be monitored periodically to determine its effectivenes, and your liver function will also be monitored. If your cholesterol and triglyceride blood levels have not been lowered to acceptable levels within three months of taking this drug, your doctor will probably discontinue its use. Before taking this drug notify your doctor if you have had a history of diabetes, peptic ulcer, or any liver or kidney disease.

For this drug to work properly, you will be placed on a special diet that restricts cholesterol and fat intake. Even if you have not had success controlling lipid levels with diets in the past, while taking this drug it is important that you faithfully stick to a low-fat regimen, reduce your weight and intake of alcoholic beverages, and exercise frequently.

Pregnancy:
Category X (see page 103).

Brand Name	Generic Name
LOPID	gemfibrozil
	(gem-FY-bro-zil)

How the Drug Works
By inhibiting the production of triglycerides (fatlike substances) and cholesterol in the liver, it reduces fat blood levels.

Purpose
Treatment of hypertriglyceridemia (Type IV hyperlipidemia).

Dosage
Adults: 600 mg twice daily taken 30 minutes before the morning and evening meals. Some patients may find a lower daily dose of 900 mg effective, while others will require as much as 1,500 mg daily.

Side Effects
Less common: Diarrhea; nausea; vomiting; gas, heartburn, or stomach upset; skin rash and itching; muscle cramps.

Adverse Reactions
Rare: Abdominal pain with nausea and vomiting, fevers and chills, sore throat, blurred vision, dizziness, tingling in hands or feet.

Drug Interaction
Increases the effectiveness of oral anticoagulants.

Overdosage
No overdosage symptoms have been established.

Comments
Lopid (gemfibrozil) is used in patients with very high blood triglyceride levels who have been unable to lower the levels by means of diets and other therapies. This drug works primarily on reducing triglyceride fats, though it may also help reduce cholesterol fat as well.

Notify your doctor if you have had a history of gallstones or gallbladder disease, or kidney or liver disease. Take the drugs 30 minutes before your morning and evening meals. For this drug to work properly, you will be placed on a special diet that restricts cholesterol and fat intake. Even if you have not had success controlling lipid levels with diets in the past, while taking this drug it is important that you faithfully stick to a low-fat regimen, reduce your weight and intake of alcoholic beverages, and exercise frequently.

If the drug continues to cause you abdominal pain, nausea, and diarrhea, notify your doctor. The drug may also cause dizziness and blurred vision. Hence, use caution if driving or operating machinery that requires alertness.

Pregnancy
Category B (see page 103).

Brand Name   *Generic Name*
MEVACOR*   lovastatin
                                   (low-va-STATE-in)

How the Drug Works

By inhibiting the action of a certain enzyme, it reduces the production of cholesterol in the body and increases the rate at which the body removes it.

Purpose

Reduction of elevated total cholesterol and LDL (low-density-lipoprotein) cholesterol levels (hypercholesterolemia), or just elevated LDL cholesterol levels. Treatment of hypertriglyceridemia.

Dosage

Adults: 20 mg once daily with the evening meal, followed by up to 80 mg daily in single or divided doses. Dose changes should be made in four-week intervals; dose levels may be influenced by the severity of the hypercholesterolemia.

Side Effects

Common: Headache.

Less common: Diarrhea; constipation; gas, heartburn, or stomach upset; skin rash and itching.

Adverse Reactions

Rare: Abdominal pain with nausea and vomiting, muscle aches or cramps, heartburn, blurred vision.

---

* A recently approved antihyperlipidemia drug, Pravachol (pravastatin), has a similar action as Mevacor: it inhibits the body's cholesterol production. The side effect and drug interaction profile of the two drugs are similar.

Drug Interaction

Increases the effectiveness of oral anticoagulants, cholestyramine, and clofibrate.

Overdosage

No overdosage symptoms have been established.

Comments

Mevacor (lovastatin) is used to lower blood levels of cholesterol in patients with primary hypercholesterolemia; "primary" means their hypercholesterolemia is not the result of another problem such as diabetes or hypothyroidism ("secondary" hypercholesterolemia). With this drug, your cholesterol blood levels should begin to decrease within the first two weeks of treatment, with maximum benefits occurring within four to six weeks. Your doctor will monitor your liver function periodically and occasionally check your eyes to measure the drug's effectiveness.

Take the drug with a meal for maximum absorption and effectiveness. For this drug to work properly, you will be placed on a special diet that restricts cholesterol and fat intake. Even if you have not had success controlling lipid levels with diets in the past, while taking this drug it is important that you faithfully stick to a low-fat regimen, reduce your weight and intake of alcoholic beverages, and exercise frequently.

If the drug gives you aching muscles, abdominal pain, nausea, or diarrhea, and the symptoms persist, notify your doctor. The drug may also cause dizziness and blurred vision, so use caution if driving or operating machinery that requires alertness.

Pregnancy

Category X (see page 103).

Brand Name	*Generic Name*
NICOLAR	niacin (nye-a-sin)
	or nicotinic
	(nik-o-TEEN-ik) acid

How the Drug Works

By reducing the production of low-density lipoproteins (cholesterol) and inhibiting the conversion of fatty tissue to cholesterol and triglycerides, it lowers blood cholesterol and triglyceride levels.

Purpose

Treatment of hyperlipidemia (elevated cholesterol and/or triglycerides).

Dosage

Adults: 250 to 200 mg three times daily, generally with or following meals.

Side Effects

Common: Feeling of warmth, tingling sensation, flushing or redness.

Less Common: Diarrhea, dizziness, dryness of skin, headache, nausea, vomiting, stomach pain.

Adverse Reactions

Abdominal pain with nausea and vomiting, persistent nausea and vomiting, yellow eyes and skin, dark-colored urine or light-colored stools (possible hepatitis), blurred vision.

Drug Interaction

Increases the effectiveness of some hypertensive drugs.

Decreases the effectiveness of some antidiabetic drugs.

Overdosage
If any of the following symptoms develop, notify your physician immediately: See adverse reactions, and also sweating, weakness, and fainting.

Comments
Niacin, or nicotinic acid, was first identified in 1937 as the food factor (or vitamin) that, if deficient, caused a "diet-deficient" disease called pellagra, whose principal early symptoms are dermatitis and diarrhea. Another, though not well established, therapeutic effect of nicotinic acid is its ability to dilate blood vessels near the surface of the skin. For this reason, some doctors may recommend the use of nicotinic acid to help improve circulation in the hands or feet. This effect also explains why people become flushed or reddish while taking the drug.

A more important issue for patients with hyperlipidemia, however, is the medicine's ability to reduce the body's production of cholesterol and triglycerides, thereby reducing blood fat levels. It is given to people who have not responded to diet or weight loss and is used primarily with other medications.

Although niacin can be purchased as a vitamin, certain strengths are available only by prescription. Treatment of hyperlipidemia with niacin should be conducted only under a doctor's supervision. Inform your doctor if you have a history of diabetes, liver disease, gout, glaucoma, or stomach ulcers.

To minimize any possible stomach irritation, take the medication with your meals. Although it is quite harmless, if you find that the flushing bothers you, one aspirin a day may reduce this effect. Your doctor may also recommend a time-release capsule that reduces excessive flushing.

For this medicine to work properly, you will be placed on a special diet that restricts cholesterol and fat intake. Even if you have not had success controlling lipid levels with diets in the past, while taking this drug it is important that you faithfully stick to a low-fat regimen, reduce your weight and intake of alcoholic beverages, and exercise frequently.

Pregnancy

Category C (see page 103). Since the drug appears in breast milk, consult your doctor before you begin breast-feeding.

Brand Name	*Generic Name*
LORELCO	probucol
	(pro-BYOO-kole)

How the Drug Works

By inhibiting the movement of cholesterol from the intestine into the bloodstream, and possibly decreasing cholesterol production in the body, it reduces blood cholesterol levels.

Purpose

Treatment of hypercholesterolemia; or hypercholesterolemia and hypertriglyceridemia.

Dosage

Adults: 250 mg twice daily, with morning and evening meals.

Side Effects

Common: Diarrhea, bloating, nausea, vomiting, stomach pain.
Less common: Headaches, dizziness, numbness or tingling in hands, feet, or face.

Adverse Reactions

Rare: Swelling of face, hands, or feet; malodorous sweating.

Drug Interaction

May decrease clofibrate's effectiveness.

Overdosage

If any of the following symptoms develop, notify your physician immediately: Loose stools, diarrhea, flatulence.

Comments

Lorelco (probucol), introduced in 1977, is less effective than some of the other lipid-lowering drugs. Hence, it is used more often in people with mild rather than severe hypercholesterolemia, and in conjunction with other lipid-lowering drugs, such as Questran (page 259) or Colestid (page 261). Let your doctor know if you have a history of gallbladder disease, gallstones, liver disease, or heart disease, especially arrhythmia.

The drug will be better absorbed if taken with your meals. For this medicine to work properly, you will be placed on a special diet that restricts cholesterol and fat intake. Even if you have not had success controlling lipid levels with diets in the past, while taking this drug it is important that you faithfully stick to a low-fat regimen, reduce your weight and intake of alcoholic beverages, and exercise frequently.

Though animal studies have not demonstrated impaired fertility or damage to the fetus, there are no adequate human studies. Therefore it is recommended for women patients who want to become pregnant to withdraw from the drug and use effective birth control for six months before they want to conceive, since the drug remains in the body for extended periods.

If the drug continues to cause diarrhea, nausea, vomiting, or stomach pain, notify your doctor. As it may also cause dizziness and blurred vision, use caution if driving or operating machinery that requires alertness.

Pregnancy

Category B (see page 103). As it is not known if this drug appears in breast milk, notify your doctor before breast-feeding.

Brand Name	*Generic Name*
CHOLOXIN	dextrothyroxine
	(dex-tro-thy-ROX-een)

How the Drug Works
By increasing the destruction of cholesterol in the liver, and increasing bile secretions (which prevents cholesterol from being absorbed into the bloodstream), it lowers blood cholesterol levels.

Purpose
Treatment of hypercholesterolemia.

Dosage
Adults: Initially 1 mg to 2 mg daily, followed by monthly increases of 1 mg to 2 mg daily, to a maximum of 4 mg to 8 mg daily.

Children: Initially 0.05 mg daily, followed by monthly increases of 0.05 mg to a maximum of 4 mg daily.

Side Effects
Less common: Nervousness, insomnia, constipation, stomach upset.

Adverse Reactions
Uncommon to rare: Heart palpitations, weight loss, unusual sweating, shortness of breath, hand tremors, fever, diarrhea, changes in menstrual cycle, leg cramps, hair loss, increased need to urinate.

Drug Interaction
Increases effects of digitalis drugs and oral anticoagulants.

Overdosage
If any of the following symptoms develop, notify your physician immediately: Chest pains, severe stomachache with nausea and vomiting, or fast or irregular heartbeat.

Comments
Choloxin (dextrothyroxine) is used to lower high blood levels of cholesterol. The drug is usually not given to people with thyroid

problems, high blood pressure, or a history of heart disease, and if so, they are closely monitored. For example, at any sign of nervousness, insomnia, or weight loss—all suggesting an overactive thyroid or hyperthyroidism—your doctor would reduce the dosage or discontinue the drug. Your doctor also needs to know if you have had a history of diabetes, or liver or kidney disease.

For this medicine to work properly, you may be placed on a special diet that restricts cholesterol and fat intake. Even if you have not had success controlling lipid levels with diets in the past, while taking this drug it is important that you faithfully stick to a low-fat regimen, reduce your weight and intake of alcoholic beverages, and exercise frequently.

Notify your doctor if you develop any heart palpitations, chest pains, diarrhea, or skin rash.

Pregnancy

Category C (see page 103). Since the drug appears in breast milk, consult your doctor before you begin breast-feeding.

CARDIAC DIARY

Date	Time	Symptoms	Trigger	Relieved by	Meds	Duration

Glossary

Anemia: a reduction in the number of red blood cells in the blood. The red blood cells contain hemoglobin, which carries the oxygen from the lungs to all parts of the body.

Aneurysm: a localized dilatation of a blood vessel or of the left ventricle.

Angina pectoris: severe chest pain originating in the middle of the chest, possibly radiating to the left shoulder and left arm, due to a temporary decreased blood supply to the heart muscle.

Angiography: an X-ray examination of the blood vessels following an injection of radiopaque material into the vessels to make them visible.

Angioplasty: *see* **PTCA.**

Angiotensin: a potent vasoconstricting hormone produced by an interaction by another hormone, renin.

Antiarrhythmics: medication that is prescribed for heart rhythm disturbances.

Anticoagulants: medication prescribed to reduce blood clotting.

Antihypertensives: medication prescribed to reduce hypertension (elevated blood pressure).

Aorta: the largest artery in the body, it arises from the left ventricle and brings oxygenated blood to the entire body.

Aortic valve: three thin pieces of tissue that form a door to separate the left ventricle from the aorta, which opens in systole to allow blood to exit into the aorta and closes in diastole to prevent blood from flowing back into the left ventricle.

Arrhythmia: an abnormal or irregular heartbeat.

Arteriosclerosis: hardening of the arteries.

Atherosclerosis: hardening of the arteries characterized by deposits of fat and cholesterol on the inner walls of blood vessels.

Atrial fibrillation: a very rapid twitching of the atrium, which creates a very rapid irregular heartbeat.

Atrium: the upper chamber of each side of the heart; the right atrium receives oxygen-poor blood returning from the body and the left atrium receives oxygen-rich blood from the lungs.

Bundle branch block: abnormal electrical conduction of the heartbeat impulse in the left ventricle creating an electrical abnormality on the ECG, or electrocardiogram.

Cardiac catheterization: a test that evaluates the function of the heart and its blood vessels by passing a long thin tube up an artery originating in the groin (femoral artery, or Judkins' approach), or right arm (brachial artery, or Sones' approach), through which pressures are measured and pictures are taken.

Cardiomyopathy: disease of the heart muscle.

Cardioversion: restoration of the normal heartbeat by electrical shock.

Carotid artery: two blood vessels—one on the left and one on the right side of the head—that are major suppliers of blood to the brain.

Cholesterol: an important steriod building block taken into the body in the form of animal food products and also manufactured by the body. There are two important components of cholesterol, LDL, or low-density lipoprotein, which deposits on the blood vessel walls and produces plaque, potentially obstructing blood flow; and HDL, high-density lipoprotein, which helps to extract cholesterol from the blood vessel walls, potentially reducing the plaque buildup.

Conduction system: the system of small electrical impulses generated spontaneously in the heart, which cause the heart muscle to contract in normal sequence.

Congenital heart disease: physical or developmental abnormalities of the heart that are inherited, or related to influences during gestation.

Congestive heart failure: an abnormal back-up of blood in the lungs and the right side of the heart due to abnormal function of the left ventricle or obstruction of blood flow, such as in mitral stenosis. The symptoms of congestive heart failure may include shortness of breath and swelling of the feet (*see* **Edema**).

Coronary arteries: the major blood vessels that arise from the aorta and supply oxygenated blood to the heart muscle. They consist of a major branch called the *left main*, which branches into two blood vessels; the *left anterior descending*, which supplies the front of the heart; the *left circumflex*, which supplies the side of the heart; and a separate blood vessel called the *right coronary artery*, which supplies the lower portion of the heart.

Coronary artery bypass surgery (CABG): an operation in which blockages in the coronary blood vessels are treated. In the procedure, pieces of vein are taken from blood vessels in the leg and are used to carry blood from the aorta to just past the coronary artery blood vessel blockage so that the muscle is supplied with oxygenated blood. Another technique involves an artery from the chest wall (left internal mammary artery, LIMA), which is very effective.

Coronary spasm (Prinzmetal's angina): A temporary cessation of the blood flow in the coronary vessel due to sudden onset of a local contraction of the blood vessel. This can occur in a normal area or where there is underlying plaque.

Cyanosis: a dark blue or purplish discoloration of the lips, nails, or fingertips due to a decrease in the oxygen content of the blood. This can be caused by congenital heart disease or severe lung disease.

Defibrillation: a technique usually involving electrical current that reverses fibrillation (rapid irregular contractions) of the heart and returns the heart rhythm to normal.

Dental prophylaxis: the taking of antibiotics before and after dental work as a special precaution against infection for patients who have underlying heart disease, particularly congenital or valvular heart disease.

Diabetes mellitus: a metabolic disease in which a deficiency of insulin in the body prevents the normal utilization of carbohydrates and sugars; it leads to elevated blood sugars and subsequent major complications.

Diastole: the time period of the cardiac cycle during which the ventricle fills with blood (just prior to systole).

Digitalis: a cardiac drug derived from the purple foxglove plant which is used to control heart rhythm disturbances and also to increase the strength of the heart muscle.

Diuretics: a specific category of drugs that promote increased excretion of urine.

Dyspnea: difficulty breathing or shortness of breath.

Echocardiography: a sound wave test that evaluates the structure and function of the heart muscle and heart valves.

Edema: an excessive accumulation of fluid in body tissues, especially the lungs (pulmonary edema) or legs (peripheral edema).

Effusion: the accumulation of excess fluid in body cavities, such as the lining of the lungs (pleural effusion) or the sac around the heart (pericardial effusion).

Electrocardiogram: a graphic recording of the intrinsic electrical activity of the heart.

Embolism: blockage of a vessel by a blood clot or infection that has traveled from another part of the body.

Endocarditis: an inflammation or infection of the lining of the heart. The term usually refers to infection of one of the heart valves.

Heart failure: *see* **Congestive heart failure.**

Hemorrhage: bleeding.

High-density lipoprotein (HDL): *see* **Cholesterol.**

Hypercholesterolemia: elevated cholesterol.

Hypertension: elevated blood pressure.

Hyperkalemia: elevated levels of potassium in the blood serum.

Hypertrophy: increase in size of an organ or part. The term frequently refers to an enlargement of the heart muscle of the left ventricle secondary to high blood pressure or aortic stenosis.

Hypokalemia: decreased levels of potassium in the blood serum.

Hypotension: decreased blood pressure.

Hypoxia: decreased oxygen in the blood.

IHSS (Idiopathic hypertrophic subaortic stenosis, or hypertrophic cardiomyopathy): a specific cardiac muscle disease in which part of the heart muscle is thickened, obstructing blood flow out of the ventricle. This disease can be inherited.

Infarction (Myocardial infarction): sudden cessation of blood flow to a muscle or organ causing its death. Myocardial infarction refers specifically to prolonged decreased oxygen supply to the heart muscle causing its localized death, which leads to a portion of subsequent scarring.

Ischemia: decreased blood supply to a specific organ.

Left atrium: upper chamber of the left side of the heart that receives oxygenated blood from the lungs and leads into the left ventricle through the mitral valve.

Left bundle branch block: specific conduction abnormality of the electrical activity of the heart as manifested on the electrocardiogram.

Left ventricle: the major pumping chamber of the heart, it receives blood from the left atrium and empties blood through the aortic valve into the aorta.

Mitral stenosis: the mitral valve leaflets become thickened and calcified, obstructing blood flow from the left atrium to the left ventricle. Usually this is due to rheumatic heart disease.

Mitral valve prolapse (MVP): specific disease of the mitral valve in which the tissues of the leaflet are redundant, or floppy, leading to the hammocking of the valve into the left atrium when it closes.

Murmur: abnormal sound of blood moving through the heart. This can be due to stenosis (poor opening) or regurgitation (poor closing) of the heart valve.

Myocardial infarction: *see* **Infarction.**

Myocarditis: inflammation of the heart muscle. Usually due to viral illness.

Myocardium: heart muscle.

Pacemaker: the specific region in the left atrium, or an artificial device that supplies the electrical stimulation causing contraction of the heart.

Pericardium: thin membrane surrounding the heart muscle.

Peripheral vascular disease: a condition affecting the blood vessels in which there is limited blood flow supply to the arms and legs. It can be manifested by cramps (claudication) of the calf muscles when walking.

Platelets: small particles circulating in the bloodstream that serve an important role in clotting and are also implicated in sudden blood vessel blockage.

Plaque: abnormal demarcation or swelling on the inner lining of an artery, usually produced by cholesterol and fat deposits.

PTCA (percutanous transluminal coronary angioplasty): the dilatation of a blocked blood vessel by the introduction of a balloon-tipped catheter that expands at the area of blockage, thereby crushing the blockage and improving blood flow.

Pulmonary edema: *see* **Edema.**

Pulmonary embolism: *see* **Embolism.**

Pulse: the rhythmic expansion of arteries due to the contraction of the heart as it sends blood through the aorta to all the blood vessels of the body. A pulse can be felt in the wrist (radial pulse) or neck (carotid pulse).

QRS complex: this specific electrocardiogram signal causes the contraction of the left ventricle.

Regurgitation: back flow, or leakage, through a heart valve.

Renin: an enzyme produced in the kidney that acts to produce angiotensin from its precursor, angiotensinogin.

Rheumatic fever: a systemic reaction to streptococcal bacterial infection, which is manifested by an inflammation in the heart, the joints, and the nervous system. This inflammation of the heart can lead to rheumatic heart disease, causing thickening and scarring of the heart valves and, particularly, mitral stenosis.

Right bundle branch block: specific electrical disturbance of the conduction in the left ventricle as seen on an electrocardiogram.

Right ventricle: the pumping chamber on the right side of the heart that receives deoxygenated blood from the right atrium through the tricuspid valve and pumps it into the pulmonary artery and the lungs through the pulmonic valve.

Shunt: an abnormal passage of blood. In an intracardiac shunt, the blood moves from the left side to the right side of the heart through a congenital hole, such as in an atrial or ventricular septal defect.

Sodium: a naturally occurring metalic element that has been implicated in exacerbating hypertension.

Stress test: an examination performed to evaluate the subject's exercise capacity. This may be performed on a treadmill—a moving surface with varying speeds and elevations; on a bicycle; with the administration of radionuclear particles (thallium); or with pharmacological agents to mimic exercise (dypiridamole or adenosine).

Sudden death: the sudden cessation of adequate circulation to the heart and brain causing a fainting spell. This is usually due to a heart rhythm disturbance. A patient can be successfully resuscitated from an episode of sudden death and undergo extensive evaluation and treatment to prevent its recurrence.

Syncope: sudden loss of consciousness; fainting.

Thrombus: a blood clot that forms in a blood vessel or in a heart chamber.

Valve: thin flaps of tissue that serve to separate the various cardiac chambers. Valves are also found in veins to prevent back flow of blood.

Varicose veins: abnormal swelling and dilatation of a vein; it can occur in the calf and appear as a bluish streak.

Veins: thin-walled blood vessels that return blood to the right side of the heart.

Index

heart blocks, 223
heart diaries. *See* cardiac diaries
heart disease
angina pectoris (*see* angina pectoris)
blood clots (*see* blood clots)
congestive heart failure (CHF) (*see* congestive heart failure)
coronary artery disease (*see* coronary artery disease)
deaths related to, xix
diagnosis of (*see* diagnostic tests)
diets and (*see* diets)
doctors and (*see* doctors)
drugs for (*see* heart drugs)
drugs that reverse, 52
endocarditis (*see* endocarditis)
general description of, 30–31
heart attacks (*see* heart attacks)
heart muscle disease, 47–48
hypertension (*see* hypertension)
mitral valve prolapse (MVP), 36–40
normal heart function, 27–30
palpitations (*see* arrhythmias)
patient attitudes toward, 6–8
patients and (*see* patients)
recovery (*see* recovery)
risk factors for (*see* risk factors)
spasms, 32
surgery for (*see* corrective procedures)
symptomless, 79–81
treatment of (*see* heart drugs; Treatments)
types of, 27–50
heart drugs. *See also* treatments
additional information about, 72–73
antiarrhythmics (*see* antiarrhythmics)

antihyperlipidemics (*see* antihyperlipidemics)
beta blockers (*see* beta blockers)
blood levels of, 59–61
blood-related (*see* blood-related drugs)
this book about, xxi–xxii
calcium antagonists (*see* calcium antagonists)
capabilities of, 51–53
combinations of, 70–71 (*see also* diuretic combinations)
diuretics (*see* diuretics)
doctor-patient issues (*see* doctors; patients)
dosage determination of, 67–71
discontinuation of, 61–62
functions of, 56–65
heart disease and (*see* heart disease)
interactions with food, 66–67
interactions with other drugs, 62–65
introduction of new, xix–xxi
listed, xiii–xviii
long-acting *vs* short-acting, 61
metabolism and, 56–57
paradoxical reactions to, 73–75
potassium supplements, 216–20
questions to ask about, 65
receptor sites and, 58–59
recording usage of (*see* cardiac diaries)
schedules of, 53–54
sharing information about, 54–56
side effects of, 71–75, 78
tolerance and, 57–58
understanding, 77–78
vasodilators (*see* vasodilators)